INTRODUCTION

Anxiety, fear, worry, and other troublesome emotional reactions are issues most of the world's population deals with. Since time immemorial, it has been a bane and a thorn in the sides of many. It is also the reason why many people have failed to live great and fulfilling lives. Many have endured lives with panic attacks, manic anxiety, and so on. For many years, these mental challenges and disorders have gone on without an antidote, however, with the advancement of neuroscience and behavioral psychology, Scientists believe they have finally found some effective answers and are now able to proffer viable solutions and tips that could help many overcome the limitations of anxiety and fear, enabling them to live fulfilling lives. The primary objective, therefore, of this book, is to provide a guide by which everyone can understand and avail themselves of the knowledge of neuroscience and use it to overcome the hurdles and roadblocks to living an anxiety free life. It is the author's hope that as many that read and implement the tenets noted in this book will be able to reconfigure their minds and not only overcome anxiety and all its vices, but experience genuine peace, joy, furthermore awesome of what life needs to offer.

CHAPTER 1
THE MEANING OF NEUROSCIENCE

Neuroscience (or neurobiology) is the study of the nervous system and brain. It is a multidisciplinary part of biology that joins physiology, molecular biology, anatomy, cytology, numerical modeling, and psychology to understand the basic and rising properties of neurons and neural circuits.

The degree of neuroscience has augmented later some an ideal opportunity to incorporate different procedures used to examine the sensory system at different scales and the cycles used by neuroscientists have expanded enormously, from nuclear and cell examinations of individual neurons to imaging of unmistakable, motor, and emotional endeavors in the cerebrum.

Neuroscience in this way assists us with bettering comprehend the mind and the sensory system. It assists us with understanding the hardware and the cycles which achieve our conduct and helps us in vanquishing the negative feelings which have so bothered our lives. The motivation behind this work, thusly, is to utilize the information found inside neuroscience as a vital aspect for opening the issues of uneasiness, dread, alarm assaults and other negative passionate responses we so frequently experience and give us an advantage in battling and defeating them.

We will currently zero in on seeing a portion of these negative feelings somewhat more, beginning with tension. All things considered, similarly as Sun Tzu said, "assuming you know your foe and know yourself, your triumph won't be in doubt"

CHAPTER 2
UNDERSTANDING ANXIETY

What is Anxiety? Anxiety is a feeling portrayed by an unsavory condition of internal disturbance, frequently joined by anxious conduct, for example, pacing to and fro, substantial protests, and rumination. It is the uniquely ghastly considerations of dread over predicted events.

Anxiety is a tendency of restlessness and stress, normally summarized and unfocused as an overcompensation to a situation that is genuinely considered undermining. It is routinely joined by solid strain, pressure, shortcoming and problems in center. At the point when nervousness is capable much of the time, the individual might encounter the evil impacts of an uneasiness problem. Uneasiness is solidly related to fear, which is a response to a certifiable danger and an abhorrence for risk. People facing uneasiness might pull back from conditions which have prompted nervousness previously.

The Difference Between Anxiety and Fear

Anxiety is like dread however the two are really unique. Nervousness can be separated from dread by perceiving that dread is a suitable, scholarly, and passionate response to an evident risk. Tension is related to the specific acts of instinctive responses, protected lead or break. Tension has frequently been clarified as "a future-centered demeanor state in which one can't or is reluctant to confront impending negative events." Another sign of nervousness is devastation, dread, or anxiety. Thusly, the genuine distinction among nervousness and dread lies in the way that tension is an antagonistic passionate response to an anticipated occasion, which may not represent any genuine danger, while dread is misgiving identified with obvious danger.

ATTRIBUTES OF ANXIETY

Anxiety can be capable for quite a while and is drawn out with regular aftereffects that decline individual fulfillment. This is known as ongoing uneasiness. It can likewise be knowledgeable about short inconsistent, undesirable mental breakdowns, known as serious tension. Manifestations of nervousness can broaden in

number, power, and repeat, dependent upon the person. While almost everyone has experienced uneasiness sooner or later in their lives, most don't foster extreme problems with tension. Nervousness might cause mental and physiological manifestations. The risk of nervousness prompts despairing and may even provoke a singular harming themselves, which is the explanation there are various 24-hour self destruction watch hotlines.

The social effects of uneasiness might make one pull out from conditions which have instigated tension or negative musings previously. Different effects might incorporate fretfulness, addition or decrease in sustenance utilization, and expanded motor tension, similar to foot tapping.

The psychological impacts of anxiety may include thoughts about speculative threats, paranoia, etc. For example, whilst the fear of death may be one which everybody has, anxiety–perhaps because of a near death experience–may cause one to fear and become apprehensive of death inordinately, even when he is clearly safe.

The physiological results of nervousness may include:

- Neurological: cerebral pain, paresthesia, fasciculations, vertigo, or presyncope
- Digestive: stomach pain, sickness, the runs, acid reflux, dry mouth, or bolus
- Respiratory: brevity of breath or murmuring relaxing
- Cardiac: palpitations, tachycardia, or chest pain
- Muscular: weariness, tremors, or tetany
- Cutaneous: sweat, or bothersome skin

TYPES OF ANXIETY

There are various types of tension. Seeing appropriately every one of these sorts of uneasiness gives you the high ground you want to defeat them. They are as follows:

<u>EXISTENTIAL ANXIETY</u>

I am certain everybody has, now and again, asked the million-dollar inquiry, "for what reason am alive?" Existential emergencies are periods when individuals question whether their lives have importance, reason, or worth. This can prompt tension, which

may be, yet not generally, joined to agony or pity. This problem of the significance and justification behind human presence is a critical point of convergence of the philosophical custom of existentialism.

The realist Søren Kierkegaard, in his book, *The Concept of Anxiety (1844)*, portrayed uneasiness or dread as the "tipsiness of opportunity" and proposed the chances for uplifting objectives of nervousness through the uncertain exercise of obligation and picking.

The researcher Paul Tillich depicted existential tension as "the state wherein a being is familiar with its conceivable nonbeing". Tillich battles that this tension can be recognized as a part of the human condition, or it might be against, in any case, with negative outcomes.

According to Viktor Frankl, the author of Man's Search for Meaning, when an individual is defied with ludicrous human dangers, the most fundamental of each human wish is to find a meaning of life to battle the "injury of nonbeing" as death is near.

Contingent upon the danger, psychoanalytic hypothesis perceives the accompanying sorts of anxiety:

- Realisti
- c
- Neuroti
  c Moral

TEST ANXIETY

We've all been there. A test is coming up, maybe in an especially troublesome region, suppose, Mathematics or history, and out of nowhere, we become extremely tense and restless. This type of nervousness is alluded to as test uneasiness. Test nervousness is a blend of physiological worry, pressure and generous signs, close by pressure and dread of frustration, that occur before or during test circumstances. It is a physiological condition where people experience ridiculous strain, nervousness, and pain during, just as in the past, taking an assessment. This nervousness makes imperative limits to learning and execution. Research shows that raised degrees of test uneasiness have a close relationship to exit rates and wretchedness among understudies. Test uneasiness can have more broad outcomes, unfavorably impacting a researcher's social, excitement, and conduct advancement.

Test tension is unavoidable among understudies. This was viewed as the case from the get-go, through research done as far back as the 1950s by experts like George Mandler and Seymour Sarason. Sarason's sibling, Irwin G. Sarason, by then added to early assessment of test uneasiness, clarifying the association between the effects of test nervousness, other focused sorts of tension, and summed up anxiety.

Test uneasiness can in like manner be named as expectant nervousness, situational nervousness or assessment tension. Some nervousness is standard and is required to remain mentally ready. Nevertheless, it can likewise achieve actual agony, inconvenience thinking, and stress. Unsatisfactory execution arises not because of insightful problems or helpless educational preparation, yet the negative sentiments that go with test nervousness causes cognitive decline and low proficiency. Specialists recommend that some place in the scope of 25-40% of understudies experience test anxiety.

Analysts accept that thoughts of anxiety occur to aid an individual in the instance of threat. Anxiety readies the body genuinely, subjectively, and behaviorally to recognize and manage danger. Thus, an individual's body starts to hyperventilate to permit more oxygen to enter the circulatory system, redirect blood to muscles, and sweat to cool the skin. The anxiety reaction in some depends on the likelihood of terrible things occurring around them and the person's capacity to adapt to them. On account of test taking, this may be a bad test grade that keeps the understudy from advancing to a higher institution, e.g. college. An individual's convictions about their own capabilities are a type of self-information, which assumes a significant job in dissecting circumstances that may be compromising. At the point when an individual has thoughts of low capability about their capacities, they are probably going to foresee negative results. Accordingly, evaluative circumstances including tests and examinations are seen as additionally threatening by students who have low competencies or simply unprepared.

Test nervousness involves of:

- Physiological anxiety – Physical signs incorporate headaches, stomach pulsates, nausea, detachment of the guts, over the top sweating, curtness of breath, daze or passing out, quick heartbeat and dry mouth. Test nervousness can in like manner brief mental episodes, in which the understudy might have an unforeseen genuine dread, inconvenience breathing, and remarkable inconvenience.

- Worry and dread – maladaptive understandings. This incorporates tragic cravings for hopelessness and destiny, dread of frustration, unpredictable musings, self-judgment, negative self-appraisal, disappointment and standing out oneself frightfully from others.

- Cognitive/Behavioral – The inability to zero in prompts ruined exhibitions on tests. Wriggling during or through the test. Understudies consistently report "blanking out" regardless of the way that they have perused satisfactorily for the test.
- Emotional – low certainty, debilitation, shock, and a considered hopelessness.

Research shows that parental assumptions is connected with test uneasiness. Different explanations behind test tension might incorporate dread of dissatisfaction, waiting, and past helpless test execution, just as, characteristics of the test condition, for instance, nature of the assessment, ventilation of the corridor, time requirements.

STRANGER ANXIETY

Stranger uneasiness is a sort of nervousness that youngsters and little children experience when introduced to pariahs or outsiders. It can happen whether or not the youngster is with a parental figure or another person they trust. It is generally common somewhere in the range of 6 and a year. It might yet likewise rehash from that point until the age of two years. As a youngster develops, uneasiness can be an issue as they blend with different kids. Kids might become hesitant to play with new kids. Cultivate youngsters are especially in danger, particularly assuming they experienced absence of care before in their life.

The nervousness a kid feels while standing up to an outcast relies upon various sensations of dread that arise in them. A few these rely upon the exercises the pariah could take. For instance, the youngster cries when going to be isolated from guardians or hurt. The dread of the obscure summons the uneasiness. Disregarding the way that uneasiness could leave in no time flat, it could likewise proceed for quite a while. As youngsters show up at two years old, their considerations of uneasiness with outcasts are practically gone. Regardless, a couple of youngsters can keep on encountering pressure up until the age of four. It is doubtful for children to experience uneasiness inside seeing a pariah in the event that it's a figure they trust, for example, their parents.

Indications of Stranger Anxiety

As shown by the University of Pittsburgh, subject to the kid, signs of more interesting nervousness can differentiate from one to kid the other. For instance;

1. Sometimes, the kid can startlingly become quiet and gaze at the pariah with fear.

2. The youngster being referred to will act hesitantly towards the untouchable, for instance clamorous crying and fastidiousness.

3. The kid will likewise cover oneself in their parent's arms or even get themselves far from the outsider by putting the parent among themselves and the stranger.

SOCIAL ANXIETY

Social nervousness is dread in friendly circumstances. A few problems related with the social uneasiness incorporate nervousness issues, disposition issues, mental imbalance range issues, dietary issues, and substance use issues. People who experience social tension will more often than not be more saved, show less presentations, and show issue with beginning and keeping up discussion. This might be because of a response to a particular social boost. Almost 90% of individuals report feeling results of social tension (for instance timidity) eventually in their lives. A big part of individuals with any friendly sensations of dread meet the standards for social tension disorder.

SOCIAL ANXIETY DISORDER

Social uneasiness issue (SAD), in any case called social dread, is a nervousness problem portrayed by a great deal of dread in no less than one social situation, causing reduced working limit and disabled social connections in certain pieces of daily existence. These sensations of dread can be initiated by evident or authentic analysis from others.

Physical incidental effects regularly incorporate over the top becoming flushed, loads of sweating, shaking, palpitations, and squeamishness. Stammering may likewise happen, close by quick talk. Mental episodes can in like manner occur under uncommon strain. A couple of victims might use alcohol or various meds to diminish fears and restraint at public gatherings.

It is fundamental for victims of social tension issue to self-cure, assuming they are unseen, untreated, or both; this can provoke alcohol enslavement, dietary problems or various kinds of substance misuse. Social uneasiness issue may

originate from dread of embarrassment or of making mistakes.

Similarly, likewise with each phobic problem, those encountering social tension as often as possible will attempt to avoid the reason for their nervousness; because of social nervousness this is especially convoluted, and in genuine cases can incite total social seclusion.

Social constitution tension (SPA) is a subtype of social uneasiness. It is focused on the evaluation of one's body by others. SPA is divided between young people, especially females.

PANIC DISORDER OR PANIC ATTACKS

Panic issue might share signs of pressure and tension, yet it is as a general rule very surprising. Alarm problem is a tension issue that happens even with next to no triggers. According to the U.S Department of Health and Human Services, this problem can be perceived by unexpected and reiterated scenes of genuine dread. Somebody who encounters this problem will in the end encounter constant, consistent dread of another event and as this development, it will begin to impact regular daily existence and an individual's overall individual fulfillment. It is represented by the Cleveland Clinic that frenzy issue impacts 2-3 percent of grown-up Americans and can begin around the time of the pre-adulthood and early grown-up years. A couple of indications incorporate upset breathing, chest torment, wooziness, shuddering or shaking, feeling faint, nausea, dread that you are letting completely go or will drop. Notwithstanding the way that they experience the evil impacts of these aftereffects during an assault, the essential incidental effect is the steady dread of having future frenzy attacks.

With alarm issue, an individual has brief episodes of outrageous trepidation and wavering, consistently put aside by shuddering, shaking, disorder, wooziness, affliction, just as breath issues. These fits of anxiety, described by the APA as dread or burden that unexpectedly arises and beat in less than ten minutes, however can proceed for quite a long time. Assaults can be invigorated by pressure, ludicrous contemplations, normal dread or dread of the obscure or even exercise. Sometimes, the trigger is muddled and the explosions can arise abruptly. To assist with thwarting an eruption, one can avoid the trigger. This being said not everything assaults can be forestalled.

Notwithstanding dreary surprising attacks of fits of anxiety, an examination of frenzy issue necessitates that said explosion have extended results: either worry

over the eruption's possible impacts, obstinate dread of future eruptions, or basic changes in activities related to the assaults. Likewise, those going through a frenzy problem experience signs even external unequivocal frenzy scenes. Habitually, regular changes in heartbeat are seen by a frenzy victim, driving them to figure something isn't right with their heart or they will have another fit of anxiety. Incidentally, an expanded cognizance (hypervigilance) of body working occurs during alarm assaults, wherein any clear physiological change is unraveled as a possibly perilous infirmity (i.e., uncommon hypochondriasis.)

STAGE ANXIETY OR PERFORMANCE ANXIETY

This type of uneasiness normally happens when an individual is approached to introduce something or to give a discourse. It is the uneasiness, dread, or strain which may set off in an individual when he requested to play out a demonstration before a gathering of individuals, whether or not it is sure or simply an idea (for example, when performing before a camera.) Acting before a horde of outsiders can cause out and out more tension than acting before known people or associates. Sporadically, anxiety in front of large audiences may be a piece of a greater illustration of social dread (social uneasiness problem), but various people experience stage tension without any broad issues. Much of the time, stage tension arises in a basic assumption for a show, regardless of whether very ahead. It has different signs: vacillating, tachycardia, quake in the hands and legs, sweat-drenched hands, facial nerve spasms, dry mouth, and discombobulation.

Stage nervousness could in any case happen in people who are even capable public speakers, just as people who are absolutely new to being before a horde of individuals. It is an exceptionally normal disorder.

As shown by a Harvard Mental Health Letter, "Tension generally has actual signs that comprises of a quick heartbeat, a dry mouth, precarious voice, becoming flushed, shaking, sweating, sickness." This happens when the body releases adrenaline into the circulatory framework getting a chain of reactions going. This response is known as the "instinctive" response, a standard cycle in the body done to safeguard itself from hurt. "The neck muscles contract, chopping the head down and perseveres, while the back muscles bring the spine into an internal curve. This, along these lines, pushes the pelvis forward and pulls the private parts up, hanging the body into an excellent fetal position."

In endeavoring to go against this position, the body will begin to shake in spots, for instance, the legs and hands. One or two things happen other than this. Muscles in the body contract, causing them to be tense and ready to attack. Second, "veins in the appendages contract". This can leave a person with the possibility of cold fingers, toes, nose, and ears. Contracted veins moreover give the body extra circulatory system to the irreplaceable organs.

Furthermore, those experiencing anxiety in front of large audiences will have a development in beat, which supplies the body with more enhancements and oxygen considering the "acute stress" driving forces. This, thusly, causes the body to overheat and perspire. Breathing will increment, so the body can get the best proportion of oxygen for the muscles and organs. This can leave the body with the effects of dry mouth, affliction, or "butterflies."

MATH ANXIETY

Engrave H. Ashcraft portrays math nervousness as "a considered strain, stress, or dread that intrudes with math execution." (2002, p. 1) The insightful examination of math nervousness begins as exactly on schedule as the 1950s, where Mary Fides Gough familiar the term mathemaphobia with portray the dread like musings of various towards science. The essential number related tension assessment scale was made by Richardson and Suinn in 1972. Since this improvement, a couple of researchers have explored math uneasiness in exploratory examinations. Hembree (1990) drove a meta-assessment of 151 examinations concerning math uneasiness. It set up that number related tension is related to helpless numerical execution on mathematical achievement tests and that number related nervousness is related to negative attitudes concerning math. Hembree also suggests that mathematical uneasiness is directly connected with math evasion.

Ashcraft (2002) suggests that significantly anxious number related understudies will avoid conditions wherein they need to perform logical assessments. Tragically, math evading achieves less ability, show, and math work later on, leaving understudies progressively anxious and mathematically unprepared to succeed. In school and school, nervous numerical understudies take less mathematical courses and will overall feel negative towards math. All things considered, Ashcraft observed that the relationship is between math nervousness and elements, for instance, sureness and motivation are solidly negative.

As shown by Schar, because math tension can cause math avoidance, an observational trouble arises. For instance, when a significantly math tense understudy performs disappointingly on a mathematical problem, it very well may be a direct result of math uneasiness, or the shortfall of ability in math because of math avoiding. Ashcraft affirmed that by running a test that ended up being continuously more mathematically testing. He saw that even significantly math-fretful individuals dominate on the principle piece of the test assessing execution. Regardless, on the last referenced and progressively problematic piece of the test, there was a more grounded negative association among precision and math anxiety.

As demonstrated by the investigation found at the University of Chicago by Sian Beilock and her gathering, math nervousness can't be connected to being horrendous at math. Right after using frontal cortex checks, analysts asserted that the assumption or translating math truly causes math uneasiness. The frontal cortex checks demonstrated that the locale of the brain that is actuated when someone has math tension covers a comparable zone of the frontal cortex where actual mischief is enrolled. Furthermore Trezise and Reeve show that understudies' numerical tension can change all through the length of a math class.

ANXIETY DISORDER

Anxiety issue are a social occasion of mental issue depicted by decisive musings of uneasiness and dread. Nervousness is a strain over future occasions, and dread is a reaction to recent developments. These feelings might cause actual aftereffects, for instance, a speedy heartbeat and unsteadiness. There are numerous uneasiness issues, including summed up nervousness problem, explicit fear, social tension issue, partition tension issue, agoraphobia, alarm issue, and particular mutism. The issue fluctuates by what brings about the indications. Individuals much of the time have more than one nervousness disorder.

The justification for uneasiness problems is accepted to be a blend of inherited and ecological elements. Hazard factors incorporate a foundation set apart by kid abuse, family heritage of mental issues, and neediness. Uneasiness problems routinely occur with other mental issues, transcendently significant burdensome issue, behavioral condition, and substance use issue. To be investigated, manifestations typically should keep going for at minimum a large portion of a year, be more than whatever may be typical for the situation, and lessen every day work. Different conditions that might achieve similar signs incorporate hyperthyroidism; coronary illness; caffeine, liquor, or pot use, and

withdrawal from explicit drugs, among others.

Without treatment, uneasiness problems will quite often remain. Treatment might incorporate routine changes, directing, and meds. Directing is normally with a type of intellectual social treatment. Meds, for instance antidepressants, benzodiazepines, or beta blockers, may improve symptoms.

About 12% of people are affected by an uneasiness issue consistently, and some place in the scope of 5-30% are impacted during their lifetime. They happen in females about twice as regularly as in guys, and as a rule emerge before 25 years. The most broadly perceived are explicit fears, which impact practically 12%, and social nervousness problem, which impacts 10%. Fears will generally impact people between the ages of 15 and 35 and turn out to be less reliable later age 55. Rates appear, apparently, to be higher in the

United States and Europe.

GENERALIZED ANXIETY DISORDER

Generalized nervousness issue (GAD) is a common problem, depicted by suffering tension which isn't focused on any one substance or situation. Those encountering summed up tension issue experience slippery persistent dread and stress and become exorbitantly upset over every day exercises. Summed up tension issue is distinguished by constant exorbitant concern combined by no less than three of the going with signs: fretfulness, weariness, redirection issues, ill humor, muscle strain, and rest aggravation. Summed up nervousness problem is the most generally perceived uneasiness issue to impact more established grown-ups. Tension can be a result of a clinical or substance misuse condition, and clinical specialists should be familiar with this. A finding of GAD is made when an individual has been amazingly anxious for a half year or more. An individual might observe that they have pressure making step by step decisions and remembering obligations due to nonattendance of obsession/interruption with stress. They regularly have a focused on appearance, with delayed sweating from the hands, feet, and axillae, and they may be crying, which can propose sadness. Before an assurance of uneasiness issue is made, specialists should preclude drug-enflamed nervousness and other clinical causes.

In youngsters, GAD may be identified with migraines, anxiety, stomach agony, and heart palpitations. Ordinarily, it begins around 8 to 9 years of age.

Specific Phobias

The single greatest arrangement of uneasiness problem is that of explicit fears which comprise all cases for which dread and tension are provoked by a specific improvement or situation. Some place in the scope of 5-12% of the general population by and large experience the evil impacts of explicit fears. Victims customarily expect terrifying outcomes from encountering the object of their dread, which can be anything from an animal to a space to a natural liquid to an unequivocal situation. Normal fears are flying, blood, water, freeway driving, and entries. Exactly when people are introduced to their fear, they might experience shaking, curtness of breath, or fast heartbeat. Individuals comprehend that their dread couldn't measure up to the genuine likely danger and simultaneously are overwhelmed by it.

AGORAPHOBIA

Agoraphobia is the specific nervousness about being in a spot or situation where retreat is extreme or embarrassing, or where help may be inaccessible. Agoraphobia is unequivocally associated with alarm issue and is routinely set off by the dread of having a fit of anxiety. A common sign incorporates needing to be in consistent perspective on an exit or other escape course. In any case the sensations of dread, the term agoraphobia is habitually used to suggest revultion rehearses that victims consistently create. For example, following a fit of anxiety while driving, someone encountering agoraphobia might foster nervousness over driving and will in this manner keep away from driving. These evasion practices can consistently have veritable results and much of the time brace the dread they are achieved by.

POST-TRAUMATIC STRESS DISORDER

Post-horrible pressure issue (PTSD) was all at once a nervousness issue (by and by moved to injury and stressor-related issues in DSM-5) that comes from an awful experience. Post-horrendous pressure can result from an outrageous situation, for instance: a battle, disastrous occasion, assault, prisoner conditions, kid misuse, tormenting, or even a deadly mishap. It can moreover come about because of enduring openness to an outrageous stressor. Normal manifestations incorporate hypervigilance, flashbacks, avoidant rehearses, uneasiness, shock and discouragement. Besides, individuals might experience rest aggravations. There are different prescriptions that structure the reason of the consideration plan for those suffering with PTSD. Such prescriptions incorporate intellectual conduct treatment (CBT), psychotherapy and backing from family and friends.

Posttraumatic stress problem (PTSD) study began with Vietnam veterans, similarly as normal and non-regular occasion losses. Studies have found the degree of contact to a ruin has been viewed as the best sign of PTSD.

SEPARATION ANXIETY DISORDER

Separation tension issue (SepAD) is the sensation of unjustifiable and unsuitable levels of nervousness over being confined from an individual or spot. Detachment uneasiness is commonplace in babies or kids, and it is exactly when this tendency is absurd or ill-advised that it will in general be considered a problem. Division nervousness issue impacts commonly 7% of grown-ups and 4% of youngsters, yet the youth cases are by and large more genuine; in specific events, even a short divergence can make alarm. Treating a youngster sooner might prevent messes. This might incorporate instructing the guardians and family on the best way to oversee it. For the most part, the guardians will incidentally support the tension since they don't have a clue how to properly manage it with the kid. Outside of parent educating and family direct, professionally prescribed prescriptions, similar to SSRIs, can be used to treat division anxiety.

SITUATIONAL ANXIETY

Situational uneasiness is achieved by new conditions or advancing occasions. It can in like manner be achieved by various occasions that make explicit people restless. Its event is astoundingly normal. Routinely, a singular will experience alarm assaults or outrageous nervousness in explicit conditions. A situation that makes one individual experience tension may not impact someone else in any way shape or form. For instance, a couple of individuals become awkward in swarms or restricted spaces, so staying in a solidly stuffed line, say at the bank or a store checkout line, may make them experience surprising nervousness, possibly a fit of anxiety. Others might experience tension when huge changes in life occur, for example, entering school, getting hitched, having youngsters, thus forth.

OBSESSIVE-COMPULSIVE DISORDER

Obsessive-impulsive turmoil (OCD) was as of late designated an uneasiness issue in the DSM-4. It is the place where the individual has insanities (alarming, persistent, and meddling musings) and driving forces (wants to on and on perform unequivocal demonstrations or customs), that are not achieved by drugs or actual problem, and which cause hopelessness or social brokenness. The conventional cycles are up close and personal standards adhered to mitigate the idea of

uneasiness. OCD impacts around 1–2% of grown-ups (a more noteworthy number of ladies than men), and less than 3% of kids and adolescents.

A person with OCD understands that the signs are unreasonable and battles against both the contemplations and the conduct. Their incidental effects could be related to outside occasions they dread (for instance, their home copying down due failing to wind down the oven) or stress that they will act unacceptably.

It is unsure why a couple of individuals have OCD, but conduct, scholarly, inherited, and neurobiological factors may be involved. Hazard factors incorporate family parentage, being single (notwithstanding the way that that might result from the issue), and higher monetary class or not being in paid work. Of those with OCD around 20% of people will beat it, and secondary effects will in any occasion decrease later some an ideal opportunity for a considerable number individuals (a further 50%.)

SELECTIVE MUTISM

Selective mutism (SM) is an issue wherein a person who is ordinarily prepared for discourse doesn't talk specifically conditions or to specific people. Specific mutism generally exists along with timidity or social uneasiness. Individuals with specific mutism stay calm regardless, when the impacts of their quietness incorporate shame, social evading, or even discipline. Specific mutism impacts around 0.8% of people eventually in their life.

Cause of Anxiety Disorders

DRUGS

Anxiety and discouragement can be achieved by substance addiction, which overall improves with postponed limitation. To be sure, even moderate, proceeded with alcohol use might expand tension levels in certain people. Caffeine, alcohol, and benzodiazepine dependence can fuel or cause uneasiness and fits of anxiety. Nervousness conventionally occurs during the exceptional withdrawal time frame from substances and can keep going for up to 2 years as a component of a post-extraordinary withdrawal problem, in with regards to a fourth of people recovering from liquor addiction. In one examination from 1988–1990, sickness in around half of patients going to passionate health organizations at one British clinical facility mental focus, for conditions including tension problem, for

model, alarm issue or social fear, was set out to be the delayed consequence of liquor or benzodiazepine dependence. In these patients, a hidden augmentation in tension occurred during the withdrawal time span followed by a suspension of their nervousness symptoms.

There is confirmation that ceaseless openness to natural solvents in the work environment can be connected with uneasiness problem. Painting, staining and floor covering laying are a part of the administrations wherein basic openings to natural solvents may occur.

Consuming caffeine might cause or build nervousness issues, including alarm issue. Those with uneasiness issue can have high caffeine affectability. Caffeine-started uneasiness issue is a subclass of the DSM-5 conclusion of substance/medication set off tension issue. Substance/drug-set off uneasiness issue falls under the class of nervousness problem, and not the order of substance-related and habit-forming messes, in spite of the way that the signs are a result of the effects of a substance.

Cannabis use is additionally related with tension issue, however the specific association between weed use and nervousness regardless of everything ought to be further investigated.

MEDICAL CONDITIONS

Sometimes, a tension issue may be an indication of a principal endocrine infection that causes sensory system hyperactivity, for instance, issues with the adrenal organ or hyperthyroidism.

STRESS

Anxiety issues can arise considering life stresses, for instance, monetary burdens, consistent actual sickness, social collaboration, nationality, or self-insight, particularly among more youthful grown-ups. Uneasiness and mental misery in midlife are risk factors for dementia and cardiovascular sicknesses during aging.

GENETICS

GAD runs in families and is regularly logical in the posterity of someone with the condition.

While tension arose as a change, in recent developments it is very normal considered unfavorably concerning nervousness problem. People with these messes have significantly delicate frameworks; thusly, their frameworks will overall get carried away to clearly harmless upgrades. On occasion, nervousness problems occur in the people who have had disturbed childhoods, displaying an expanded transcendence of tension when it appears to be a youngster will have an inconvenient future. In these cases, the nervousness arises as a way to deal with anticipate that the individual's condition will continue to introduce dangers.

PERSISTENCE OF ANXIETY

At a low level, uneasiness is certifiably not something awful. Without a doubt, the hormonal response to tension has created as a benefit, as it urges individuals to react to risks. Investigators in extraordinary prescription acknowledge that this change licenses individuals to recognize there is a possible risk and to act suitably to ensure most conspicuous possibility of protection. It has truly been exhibited that those with low levels of uneasiness have a more genuine risk of death than those with typical levels. This is because the absence of dread can bring about more prominent injury or demise. Also, patients with both nervousness and melancholy were found to have preferable wellbeing over those with discouragement alone. The compelling ramifications of the indications related with uneasiness incorporates more noticeable sharpness, speedier basis for action, and diminished probability of missing dangers. In the wild, vulnerable individuals, for example the people who are hurt or pregnant, have a lower edge for nervousness response, making them more ready. This shows a broad formative history of the nervousness reaction.

EVOLUTIONARY MISMATCH

It has been speculated that high tension is a reaction to how the social condition has changed from the Paleolithic time frame. For example, in the Stone Age there was more conspicuous skin-to-skin contact and more noteworthy consideration of newborn children by their mothers, the two of which are strategies that reduce tension. Moreover, there is more noticeable joint effort with outcasts right presently went against to affiliations only between warm families. Examiners say that the shortfall of consistent social correspondence, especially in the beginning phases, is a driving justification behind high speeds of anxiety.

Numerous current cases are presumably going to have come about as a result of a transformative bungle, which has been plainly named a "psychopathic confound." In developmental terms, a befuddle happens when an individual has characteristics that were adapted to a space that changes from the person's

current condition. For example, notwithstanding the way that a tension reaction might have been progressed to assist with dangerous conditions, for extraordinarily honed individuals in Westernized social orders essentially hearing horrendous news can motivate a strong reaction.

A formative perspective might give information into choices rather than current clinical treatment methodologies for nervousness issue. Simply understanding some uneasiness is important may facilitate a part of the frenzy related with delicate conditions. A couple of researchers acknowledge that, on a fundamental level, tension can be mediated by diminishing a patient's tendency of helplessness and a while later changing their assessment of the situation.

Anxiety can be either a current second "state" or a long haul "characteristic". However quality uneasiness addresses worrying about future occasions, tension problem is a get-together of mental issue depicted by considerations of nervousness and fear.

CO-MORBIDITY

Anxiety issues often happen with other mental prosperity issues, particularly huge burdensome issue, bipolar turmoil, dietary issues, or certain person issue. It moreover consistently occurs with character qualities, for instance, neuroticism. This investigated co-occasion is for the most part because of genetic and normal effects divided among these properties and anxiety.

Anxiety is consistently capable by those with over the top enthusiastic issue and is an intense presence in alarm disorder.

CHAPTER 3
UNDERSTANDING OTHER NEGATIVE EMOTIONAL REACTIONS

Shyness

Shyness (likewise called **diffidence**) is the feeling of trepidation, absence of solace, or clumsiness, particularly when an individual is around others. This regularly happens in new circumstances or with new individuals. Shyness can be an attribute of individuals who have low confidence. More grounded types of shyness are normally alluded to as social anxiety or social phobia. The essential attribute for shyness is a largely self-image driven fear of what others will think about an individual's conduct. These results in an individual getting terrified of doing or saying what they need to out of fear of negative responses, being giggled at, mortified or belittled, criticized or dismissed. A shy individual may just decide to keep away from social conditions all things considered.

One huge piece of timidity is social abilities improvement. Schools and guardians may surely acknowledge kids who are totally fit for feasible social joint effort. Social fitness preparing isn't given any power (difference to perusing and composing) and in this manner, bashful understudies are not permitted an opportunity to develop their ability to check out class and interface with peers. Educators can show social capacities and posture requests in a less quick and terrifying manner in order to delicately encourage timid understudies to make some commotion in class, and warm up to other children.

The fundamental justification for bashfulness contrasts. Scientists acknowledge that they have observed innate data supporting the theory that modesty is, at any rate, fairly hereditary or inheritable. In any case, there is additionally proof that proposes the climate wherein an individual is raised can in like manner be answerable for their bashfulness. This incorporates youngster misuse, particularly mental abuse, for instance, judgment. Timidity can start later an individual has experienced an actual uneasiness reaction; at various occasions, bashfulness seems to develop first and subsequently causes actual results of tension. Timidity differs from social nervousness, which is a more

broad, despondency related state of mind including the experience of dread, anxiety, or worrying about being evaluated by others in friendly conditions to the level of inciting panic.

Shyness might begin from inherited qualities, the climate wherein an individual is raised, and individual encounters. Timidity may likewise be a character attribute or can occur at explicit periods of headway in children.

CAUSES OF SHYNESS
GENETICS AND HEREDITY

Shyness is often seen as a square to people and their improvement. The justification for modesty is often addressed at this point it is found that dread is positively related to bashfulness, suggesting that horrendous youngsters are fundamentally more inclined to being tentative rather than kids less repulsive. Timidity can in like manner be seen on a characteristic level as a result of a wealth of cortisol. Exactly when cortisol is free in more imperative sums, it is known to cover an individual's invulnerable system, making them more defenseless to illness and sickness. The inherited characteristics of bashfulness are a tiny region of exploration that has been tolerating far less proportions of thought, notwithstanding the way that papers on the natural bases of modesty return to 1988. Some investigation has shown that modesty and animosity are associated through long and short kinds of the quality DRD4, but fundamentally more exploration on this is required. Further, it has been suggested that modesty and social fear (the separation between the two is getting never-endingly murky) are related to fanatical enthusiastic problem. Also, likewise with various examinations of lead in social hereditary qualities, the examination of bashfulness is caught with the amount of qualities related with, and the disorder in describing, the aggregate. Naming the aggregate – and translation of terms among hereditary qualities and brain research — in like manner causes disorders.

Fear

Fear is an inclination actuated by obvious danger or risk, which causes physiological changes and at last friendly changes, for instance, avoiding, concealing, or freezing from evident horrendous setbacks. Dread in people might happen as a result of a particular lift occurring in the present, or in assumption or longing for a future peril considered a danger to oneself. The fear

response rises up out of the impression of hazard inciting standoff with or escape from/evading the risk (in any case called the instinctive response), which in incredible occurrences of dread (ghastliness and dread) can be a freeze response or loss of motion.

In people and creatures, dread is changed by the methodology of discernment and learning. In this manner dread is chosen as levelheaded or fitting, or silly or unseemly. A nonsensical dread is known as a phobia.

Fear is immovably connected with the feeling tension, which occurs as the outcome of risks that are believed to be capricious or unavoidable. The dread reaction serves perseverance by prompting fitting behavior responses, so it has been secured all through advancement. Sociological and hierarchical exploration similarly suggests that individuals' misgivings are not only dependent on their inclination yet rather are moreover shaped by their social relations and culture, which control their understanding of when and how much dread to feel.

Numerous physiological changes in the body are connected with dread, dense as the instinctive response. An inherent response for adjusting to hazard, it works by enlivening the breathing rate (hyperventilation), beat, vasoconstriction of the fringe veins inciting becoming flushed and expanding muscle pressure including the muscles attached to each hair follicle causing "goosebumps", or even more clinically, piloerection (making a cold individual more smoking or an alarmed creature look progressively undermining), sweating, expanded blood glucose (hyperglycemia), expanded serum calcium, increase in white platelets called neutrophilic leukocytes, sharpness provoking rest irritation and "butterflies in the stomach" (dyspepsia). This rough framework might empower a daily existence structure to manage by either escaping or doing combating the risk. With the course of action of physiological changes, the mindfulness understands a feeling of fear.

The capacity to fear is a piece of human intuition. Various investigations have found that particular sensations of dread (for instance creatures, statures) are significantly more average than others (for instance blossoms, fogs.) These sensations of dread are moreover less complex to impel in the exploration office. This wonder is known as readiness. Since early individuals that raced to fear unsafe conditions will undoubtedly suffer and rehash readiness is estimated to be a genetic effect that is the eventual outcome of regular selection.

From a transformative brain science perspective, different sensations of dread may be different changes that have been useful in our developmental past. They might have made during different time spans. A couple of sensations of dread, for instance, dread of statures, may be fundamental to all warm blooded animals and made during the Mesozoic time period. Various sensations of dread, for instance, dread of snakes, may be typical to all simians and made during the Cenozoic time span. Still others, for instance, dread of mice and bugs, may be exceptional to individuals and made during the paleolithic and Neolithic time frames (when mice and bugs became huge carriers of sicknesses and damaging for crops and put away foods.)

LEARNED FEAR

Animals and people work on express sensations of dread due to learning. This has been moved in brain research as dread molding, beginning with John B. Watson's 'Little Albert' research in 1920, which was propelled directly following watching a youngster with an irrational dread of canines. A short time later, the 11-month-old youngster was formed to fear a white rat in the exploration office. The dread got summarized to incorporate other white, finished things, for instance, a hare, canine, and surprisingly a wad of cotton.

Fear can be learned by experiencing or watching a frightening terrible incident. For example, assuming a youngster falls into a well and battles to get out, the individual might develop a dread of wells, statures (acrophobia), encased spaces (claustrophobia), or water (aquaphobia). There are investigates investigating districts of the mind that are impacted by dread. When investigating these areas, (for instance, the amygdala), it was suggested that a singular sort out some way to fear whether or not they personally have experienced injury, or then again assuming they have watched the dread in others. In an examination wrapped up by Andreas Olsson, Katherine I. Approaching and Elizabeth
A. Phelps, the amygdala was impacted both when subjects watched someone else being submitted to an aversive event, understanding that a comparable treatment expected themselves, and when subjects were thusly placed in a dread instigating circumstance. This proposes dread can make in the two conditions, not simply from individual history.

Fear is affected by social and verifiable setting. For example, during the 20th century, various Americans dreaded polio, a disease that can cause passing. There are a wide range of ways that people can respond to fear. Show rules impact how probable people are to convey the

superficial presentation of dread and various sentiments. Sensations of dread could be moreover impacted by sexual character. Research has exhibited individuals from each sex had the choice to see the superficial presentation of dread essentially ideal on a male face over a female face. Females moreover saw dread generally better compared to guys. Dread of abuse is a component of saw peril and seriousness.

THE MECHANICS OF FEAR

Strange or unreasonable dread is achieved by regrettable thinking (stress) which rises out of uneasiness with a theoretical sensation of hesitation or dread. Silly dread offers a regular neural pathway with various fears, a pathway that interfaces with the sensory system to enact in essence assets if there should be an occurrence of risks or hazard. Various people are terrified of the "obscure". This silly dread can spread out to various domains, For instance, the extraordinary past, the following ten years, or even tomorrow. Unremitting silly dread has pernicious effects since the elicitor boost is routinely absent or seen from fantasizes. Such dread can make comorbidity with the tension problem umbrella. Being terrified may make people experience hopeful dread of what might lie ahead as opposed to organizing and evaluating for what might occur. For instance, "continuation of academic learning" is seen by various teachers as a risk that might cause them dread and stress, and they would like to prepare things they've been instructed than continue to examine new things. That can provoke practices, for example, inactivity and procrastination.

The vulnerability of conditions that will overall be questionable and whimsical can make nervousness more normal than other mental and actual problems in specific masses; especially the people who attract it consistently, for example, in war-ridden places or in spots of conflict, mental fighting, misuse, etc. Helpless youngster raising that gives dread can similarly disable a kid's psychological headway or character. For example, guardians exhort their youngsters not to talk with untouchables to get them. In school they would be convinced to not show dread in talking with outcasts, yet to be conclusive and moreover aware of the risks and the encompassing where it occurs. Ambiguous and mixed messages like this can impact their certainty and confidence. Scientists express talking with untouchables isn't something to be blocked at this point allowed in a parent's quality whenever required. Fostering a sensation of quietness to bargain with

various conditions is regularly upheld as a solution for nonsensical dread and as an essential fitness by different outdated techniques for reasoning.

Species-express guard responses (SSDRs) or aversion learning in nature is the specific tendency to avoid explicit risks, it is the means by which animals get by in nature. People and creatures both proposition these species-explicit guard reactions, for instance, the flight-or-battle, which moreover incorporate pseudo-hostility, phony or threatening animosity, and freeze response to risks, which is obliged by the thoughtful sensory system. These SSDRs are adapted quickly through friendly communications between others of comparative species, various species, and relationship with the climate. These acquired arrangements of reactions or responses are not entirely obvious. The creature that suffers is the creature that most certainly perceives what to dread and how to avoid this danger. A model in individuals is the reaction to seeing a snake, many jump in reverse before mentally recognizing what they are jumping away from, and periodically it is a stick rather than a snake.

Likewise, with various components of the brain, there are various spaces of the frontal cortex drew in with deciphering dread in individuals and other nonhuman species. The amygdala confers the two headings between the prefrontal cortex, nerve center, the tangible cortex, the hippocampus, thalamus, septum, and the brainstem. The amygdala expects a critical occupation in SSDR, for instance, the ventral amygdalofugal, which is essential for cooperative learning, and SSDRs are learned through association with the climate and others of comparable species. An enthusiastic response is made basically later the signs have been moved between the different districts of the frontal cortex and sanctioning the smart sensory systems; which controls the flight, battle, freeze, dread, and shut down reaction. Regularly a hurt amygdala can cause handicap in the affirmation of dread. This block can make different species miss the mark on the sensation of dread, and routinely can end up being unreasonably sure, facing greater companions, or moving toward savage animals.

Robert C. Bolles (1970), a specialist at University of Washington, needed to comprehend species-explicit protection responses and aversion learning among various creatures, and observed that the hypotheses of evasion learning and the gadgets that were used to allocate this tendency were out of touch

with the ordinary world. He theorized the species-explicit guard response (SSDR). There are three sorts of SSDRs: flight, battle (pseudo-animosity), or freeze. To be sure, even subdued animals have SSDRs, and in those minutes it is seen that animals return to atavistic standards and become "wild" again. Dr. Bolles states that responses are routinely dependent on the stronghold of a wellbeing signal, and not the aversive formed lifts. This security sign can be a wellspring of info or even improvement change. Inborn analysis or data starting from inside, muscle jolts, and uplifted heartbeat, are accepted to be more huge in SSDRs than outward information, overhauls that begins from the external condition. Dr. Bolles observed that most creatures have some regular game plan of fears, to assist with ensuring endurance of the species. Rodents will escape from any disturbing occasion, and pigeons will fold their wings harder when compromised. The wing rippling in pigeons and the dispersed running of rodents are seen as species-explicit safeguard responses or practices. Bolles acknowledged that SSDRs are shaped through Pavlovian molding, and not operant molding; SSDRs rise up out of the connection between the biological improvements and negative occasions. Michael S. Fanselow drove an assessment, to test some specific guard reactions, he saw that rodents in two particular shock conditions responded surprisingly, considering instinct or wary topography, instead of coherent information

Species-explicit safeguard reactions are made from dread and are major for endurance. Rodents that show no evasion learning, or a shortfall of dread, will as often as possible approach little cats and be eaten. Creatures use these SSDRs to continue to live, to assist with expanding their chance of wellbeing, by suffering long enough to imitate. Individuals and creatures, the equivalent have made dread to perceive what should be avoided, and this dread can be learned through relationship with others in the organization, or learned through near and dear contribution in an animal, species, or conditions that should be dodged. SSDRs are a transformative change that have been found in various species generally through the world including rodents, chimpanzees, grassland canines, and even people, a change made to empower individual creatures to manage in an unpleasant world.

Fear learning changes over the lifetime on account of trademark developmental changes in the cerebrum. This incorporate changes for the prefrontal cortex and the amygdala.

NEUROCIRCUIT IN MAMMALS

- The thalamus accumulates tangible data from the senses
- Sensory cortex gets data from the thalamus and unravels it
- Sensory cortex makes data for spread to the nerve center (acute stress), amygdalae (dread), hippocampus (memory)

The frontal cortex structures that are the point of convergence of most neurobiological occasions related with dread are the two amygdalae, arranged behind the pituitary organ. Each amygdala is a piece of an equipment of dread learning. They are essential for fitting change in accordance with pressure and express adjustments of enthusiastic learning memory. Inside seeing a compromising improvement, the amygdalae produce the arrival of chemicals that effect dread and hostility. When a response to the update of dread or antagonism begins, the amygdalae may inspire the appearance of chemicals into the body to put the person into a state of status, where they are ready to move, run, battle, etc. This careful response is overall insinuated in physiology as the instinctive response constrained by the nerve center, some piece of the limbic framework. When the individual is in test mode, inferring that there are never again any potential risks incorporating them, the amygdalae will send this data to the clinical prefrontal cortex (mPFC) where it is taken care of for near future conditions, which is known as memory consolidation.

A piece of the chemicals needed during the state of acute stress incorporate epinephrine, which controls heartbeat and processing similarly as augmenting veins and air sections, norepinephrine expanding heartbeat and circulatory system to muscles and the appearance of glucose from energy stores, and cortisol which assembles glucose, increases streaming neutrophilic leukocytes and calcium among other things.

After a situation which makes dread happens, the amygdalae and hippocampus record the event through synaptic pliancy. The prompting to the hippocampus will make the singular review various particulars including the circumstance. Pliancy and memory advancement in the amygdala are made by authorization of the neurons in the region. Test data supports that synaptic flexibility of the neurons provoking the equal amygdalae occurs with dread molding. incidentally, this designs ceaseless dread responses, for example,

posttraumatic stress problem (PTSD) or a fear. X-ray and fMRI filters have exhibited that the amygdalae not really set in stone to have such issues including bipolar or alarm issue are greater and wired for a more raised degree of fear.

A couple of frontal cortex structures other than the amygdalae have moreover been believed to be authorized when individuals are given unfortunate versus unbiased appearances, specifically the occipitocerebellar locales including the fusiform gyrus and the below average parietal/transcendent temporary gyri. Unfortunate eyes, sanctuaries and mouth appear to autonomously reproduce these brain reactions. Investigations of researchers from Zurich consider show that the chemical oxytocin related to tension and sex lessens development in your cerebrum dread center.

HOW TO HANDLE FEAR

<u>PHARMACEUTICAL</u>

A medication treatment for dread molding and fears through the amygdalae is the utilization of glucocorticoids. In one examination, glucocorticoid receptors in the central centers of the amygdalae were upset in order to all the almost certain comprehend the frameworks of dread and dread molding. The glucocorticoid receptors were prevented using lentiviral vectors containing cre-recombinase implanted into mice. Results showed that aggravation of the glucocorticoid receptors prevented restrained dread conduct. The mice were presented to sound-related signs which made them freeze regularly. In any case, a reduction of freezing was found in the mice that had stifled glucocorticoid receptors.

PSYCHOLOGY

Cognitive conduct treatment has been successful in assisting people with vanquishing their dread. Since dread is more muddled than just ignoring or eradicating recollections, a working and successful procedure incorporates people at least a few times facing their feelings of trepidation. By going toward their sensations of dread in a secured way an individual can smother the "dread initiating recollections" or stimuli.

Exposure treatment has known to have expanded to 90% of people with explicit fears to basically decrease their dread over time.

Another psychological treatment is deliberate desensitization, which is a sort of lead treatment used to absolutely kill the dread or produce a nauseated

response to this dread and override it. The replacement that happens will loosen up and will occur through molding. Through molding drugs, muscle tensioning will diminish, and breathing strategies will help in de-tensioning.

Worry

Worry insinuates the contemplations, pictures, sentiments, and exercises of a negative sort in an excess, wild way that results from a proactive mental peril assessment made to avoid or comprehend anticipated possible risks and their potential consequences.

Psychologically, stress is a piece of Perseverative Cognition (a total term for diligent considering of adverse occasions previously or later on). As an inclination "stress" is capable from tension or worry about a veritable or envisioned issue, often close to home issues, it's a trademark response to anticipated future issues. Inordinate concern is a fundamental expressive part of summed up nervousness problem. By far most experience short time frames of pressure in their lives without event; certainly, a smooth proportion of pushing has valuable results, assuming it prompts people to leave nothing to chance (e.g., appending their seat strap or buying insurance) or avoid perilous practices (e.g., enraging hazardous animals, or hitting the container hard), but with pointless disturbing people they misjudge future dangers in their examinations and in its cutoff points will overall enhance the situation as a halt which results stress.

CHAPTER 4
UNDERSTANDING ANXIETY
THROUGH NEUROSCIENCE

Anxiety, it appears, is surrounding us. There are two totally different ways that anxiety starts: through what we consider, and through responses to our condition. This is on the grounds that anxiety can be started by two entirely unexpected domains of the human brain: the cortex and the amygdala. This understanding is the eventual outcome of significant length of examination in a field known as neuroscience, which is the investigation of the design and limit of the sensory system, including the brain.

The essential model above addresses the basic rule of this book: two separate pathways in the psyche can offer rising to nervousness, and each pathway ought to be perceived and treated still up in the air help (Ochsner et al. 2009). In that model, uneasiness was mixed in the cortex pathway by contemplations of the risks of leaving the oven on for the duration of the day. Everyone is good for experiencing uneasiness through the two pathways. A couple of individuals might see that their uneasiness arises more regularly in one pathway than the other. As you'll come to see, seeing the two pathways and managing each in the most ideal way is fundamental. The inspiration driving this book is to explain the differentiations between the two pathways, show how tension is made in each, and give you reasonable ways to deal with change circuits in each pathway to make nervousness less significantly a load in your life. We'll show you how you can truly change the pathways to you with the objective that they're less disposed to make anxiety.

Analyzing the Parts of Our Brain That Deal With Anxiety

Anxiety is a complex passionate response that resembles dread. Both rise out of similar cerebrum cycles and cause practically identical physiological and direct reactions; both beginning in portions of the psyche planned to empower all animals to oversee risk. Dread and uneasiness change in that dread is regularly associated with an indisputable, present, and conspicuous risk, while nervousness occurs without prompt danger. By the day's end, we feel dread when we truly are in a tough spot—like a when a truck crosses the middle

line and heads toward us. We feel tension when we have a sensation of disappointment or distresses while we aren't, by then, in mischief's way.

Everybody encounters dread and nervousness. Occasions can cause us to feel at risk, for instance, when a hazardous rainstorm shakes our home or when we see a particular canine skipping toward us. Nervousness arises when we worry about the prosperity of a companion or relative who's quite far from home, when we hear a strange disturbance late around evening time, or when we consider all that we need to complete before a best in class cutoff time for work or school. Various people feel anxious consistently, especially when under tension. Messes start, regardless, when nervousness upsets critical pieces of our lives. Taking everything into account, we need to find out with regards to our nervousness and recover control. We need to perceive how to oversee it, so it never again limits our lives.

Anxiety can control people's lives in critical ways—a large number of which may not give off an impression of being a result of uneasiness. For example, while a couple of individuals are tormented by stresses that hit each waking second, others might believe that it's difficult to shake off. Some might gain some hard experiences branching out from home, while for other people, a dread of public talking might sabotage their movement. Another mother might have to complete a movement of schedules for a serious long time each prior day she can leave her kid with a sitter. A high schooler may be upset by terrible dreams and get suspended for battling in school later his home has been wrecked by a cyclone. A jack of all trades' uneasiness about encountering gigantic insects might reduce his compensation to a level that won't support his family. A youngster may be reluctant to go to class and hesitant to banter with her educators, undermining her training.

Despite the way that nervousness can deny a person of the ability to complete an impressive part of the fundamental activities of life, these people can return to survey every second for the duration of day to day existence. They can comprehend the justification behind their difficulties and begin to find conviction again. This arrangement is possible appreciation to a continuous learning in data about the psyche structures that make anxiety.

In the past twenty years, research on the neurological establishments of uneasiness have been coordinated in a scope of examination offices all over the planet (Dias et al. 2013). Research on creatures has uncovered new bits of knowledge with respect to the neurological foundations of dread. Structures in the mind that recognize risks and start protective responses have been recognized.

Simultaneously, new developments like useful attractive reverberation imaging and positron outflow tomography examines have given point by point data concerning how the human cerebrum responds in a grouping of conditions. When investigated, separated, and merged, this rising data licenses neuroscientists to make relationship between creature examination and human exploration. Along these lines, they are at present able to gather a clear picture of the explanations behind dread and uneasiness, giving an agreement that outperforms our understanding of any remaining human feelings.

This investigation has uncovered something huge: two really separate pathways in the cerebrum can make nervousness. One way begins in the cerebral cortex, the gigantic, tangled, faint of the cerebrum, and incorporates our perceptions and contemplations about conditions. Different endeavors even more directly through the amygdala's, two little, almond-formed designs, one on each side of the mind. The amygdala triggers the primitive instinctive response, which has been passed down practically unaltered from the underlying vertebrates on earth.

The two pathways expect a job in tension, but a couple of kinds of uneasiness are more associated with the cortex, while others can be credited to the amygdala. In psychotherapy for tension, thought has typically been based on the cortex pathway, using accommodating techniques that incorporate changing musings and battling insightfully against uneasiness. Regardless, a creating gathering of exploration proposes that the occupation of the amygdala ought to in like manner be perceived to develop a logically finish picture of how uneasiness is made and how it will in general be controlled. In this book, we'll explore the two pathways to provide you with a full picture of tension and how to change it, whatever its initiation is.

THE CORTEX AND THE AMYGDALA

Odds are you're currently familiar with the cortex, the fragment of the mind that fills the most elevated piece of the skull. It is the thinking part about the cerebrum, and some say it's the piece of the mind that makes us human since it enables us to reason, develop language, and take part in complex theory, for instance, rationale and number juggling. Species that have bigger cerebral cortices are as often as possible suspected to be more shrewd than other animals.

Ways to manage treating nervousness that attention on the cortex pathway are different and regularly focus on insight, the psychological term for the

mental cycles that by far most imply as "thinking." Thoughts beginning in the cortex may be the justification for uneasiness, or they might have the effect of expanding or reducing anxiety.

In certain occasions, changing our drugs can help us with holding our mental cycles back from beginning or adding to anxiety.

Up to this point, prescriptions for tension were less disposed to ponder the amygdala pathway. The amygdala is little; notwithstanding, it's contained a large number of circuits of cells committed to different purposes. These circuits sway love, sexual direct, shock, ill will, and dread. The occupation of the amygdala is to attach passionate importance to conditions or protests and to outline enthusiastic recollections. Those sentiments and passionate recollections can be positive or negative. In this text, we will focus on the way in which the amygdala joins uneasiness to encounters and gains nervousness delivering experiences. This will help you with understanding the amygdala so you can sort out some way to change its hardware to restrict anxiety.

We people aren't purposefully aware of the way where the amygdala interfaces uneasiness to conditions or articles, likewise as we aren't intentionally aware of the liver supporting processing. Regardless, the amygdala's enthusiastic molding influences our direct. As we'll elaborate in this review, amygdala is at the actual heart of where the tension reaction is conveyed. In spite of the way that the cortex can begin or add to tension, the amygdala is needed to trigger the nervousness response. This is the explanation a thorough method for managing watching out for nervousness requires overseeing both the cortex pathway and the amygdala pathway.

NEUROPLASTICITY

In the past twenty years, research has uncovered that the psyche has an astonishing level of neuroplasticity, which implies an ability to change its constructions and patch up its methods of reacting. For sure, even pieces of the cerebrum that were once thought hard to change in grown-ups are prepared for being adjusted, revealing that the brain truly has an astounding capacity to change (Pascual-Leone et al. 2005). For example, people whose personalities are hurt by strokes can be told to use different bits of the frontal cortex to move their arms (Taub et al. 2006). In explicit circumstances, circuits in the psyche that are used for vision can develop the capacity to respond to sound in a few days (Pascual-Leone and Hamilton 2001).

New association in the mind consistently make in amazingly fundamental habits: practice has been seemed to progress broad advancement in neurotransmitters (Cotman and Berchtold 2002). In some exploration, simply contemplating taking certain activities, such as tossing a ball or playing a tune on the piano, can cause changes in the zone of the cerebrum that controls those developments (Pascual-Leone et al. 2005). Moreover, certain drugs advance turn of events and changes in circuits of the frontal cortex

(Drew and Hen 2007), especially when gotten together with psycho-treatment. Moreover, psychotherapy alone has been seemed to make changes (Linden 2006), diminishing incitation in one zone and expanding it in others.

Unmistakably, the frontal cortex isn't fixed and unchangeable, as many individuals once expected. The circuits of your frontal cortex aren't settled absolutely by genetic characteristics; they're moreover molded by your encounters and the way wherein you think and continue. You can upgrade your cerebrum to respond out of the blue, paying little mind to what age you are. There are limits, yet then again there's an astounding level of flexibility and potential for change in your frontal cortex, including changing its tendency to make perilous levels of anxiety.

We'll help you with using neuroplasticity, close by a perception of how the cortex and amygdala pathways work, to carry out suffering upgrades in your psyche. You can use this data to change your frontal cortex's equipment with the objective that it goes against uneasiness, rather than making it.

We want to start this part with an assurance that all that we edify you in regards to the psyche right now significant, rational data that will illuminate the explanations behind nervousness and help you with perceiving how to change your cerebrum to reduce your experience of tension. We won't present unequivocal, specific depictions of the multitude of neurological cycles required; rather, we will give a straightforward, principal clarification of nervousness in the psyche that can help you with understanding the reason why certain philosophies will help you with controlling your anxiety.

If you don't know the first thing what causes your tension, you are unsuspecting when you endeavor to change it. Nervousness is made by the frontal cortex and wouldn't occur without the responsibilities of unequivocal psyche locales. Also remembering that the frontal cortex is a particularly unpredictable, interconnected structure, a great deal of which remains a riddle. There are furthermore techniques you

can use to zero in on these specific nerves that will help you with being progressively reasonable in directing or hindering the nervousness you feel.

As referred to in the show, the essential spot of uneasiness in the frontal cortex are two neural pathways that can begin a tension response. The cortex pathway is the one a large number individuals consider when they ponder the explanations behind uneasiness. You'll adapt significantly more with regards to the human cerebral cortex in the accompanying region. Until additional notification, we'll basically express that the cortex is the pathway of sensations, considerations, reasoning, imaginative psyche, intuition, insightful memory, and orchestrating. Nervousness treatment routinely centers around this pathway, probable because it's an inexorably insightful pathway, inferring that we will overall be logically aware of what's happening right currently have more admittance to what this piece of the frontal cortex is remembering and focusing on. Assuming you see that your brain keeps on going to musings that expansion your nervousness, or that you focus on questions, become occupied with stresses, or slow down in endeavoring to consider deals with any consequences regarding messes, you're in all likelihood experiencing cortex-based anxiety.

The amygdala pathway, of course, can have the incredible actual effects that uneasiness has on the body. The amygdala's different relationship with various bits of the frontal cortex license it to initiate a grouping of genuine reactions quickly. In less than a 10th of a second, the amygdala can give a surge of adrenaline, increase circulatory strain and heartbeat, make muscle pressure, and anything is possible from that point. The amygdala pathway doesn't convey contemplations that you're aware of, and it works more quickly than the cortex can. Thusly, it makes various pieces of an uneasiness response without your discerning data or control. Assuming you have an inclination that your tension has no undeniable explanation and doesn't look good, you're for the most part experiencing the effects of nervousness arising out of the amygdala pathway. Your knowledge of the amygdala is likely going to be established on your experience of its effects on you—specifically genuine changes, dread, expecting to dodge a particular situation, or having strong motivations.

Specialists consistently don't discuss the amygdala while treating uneasiness issue, which is astounding, considering that most encounters of dread, tension, or frenzy arise on account of relationship of the amygdala. Regardless, when the cortex is the loaded with on restless reasoning, the amygdala causes the actual ruckuses of tension to occur, including beating heart, sweat, muscle

pressure, etc. Nonetheless, when family specialists and therapists are endorsing drugs to diminish anxiety, they're frequently centered around the amygdala, despite the fact that they may not make reference to it by name. These prescriptions, for example, Xanax (alprazolam), Ativan (lorazepam), and Klonopin (clonazepam), regularly have the impact of quieting the amygdala.

Such steadying medications are especially reaIn this waynable at quickly reducing tension. Appallingly, they never really change the hardware of the amygdala. So, while they diminish the uneasiness response, they don't assist with changing the amygdala in habits that would be advantageous in the long run.

The amygdala has various limits that aren't related to tension, and we won't jump into them here. To comprehend the amygdala's occupation in tension, it's basic to understand that as you approach your day, the amygdala sees sounds, sights, and occasions notwithstanding the way that you may not be purposely based on them. The amygdala is looking out for anything that might exhibit expected mischief. Assuming it recognizes likely hazard, it sets off the dread response, an alarm in the body that guarantees us by setting us up to battle or escape.

Think of it as thusly: we are the genealogies of unfortunate people. Early individuals whose amygdala reacted to likely hazards and made a strong dread response were well headed to carry on in cautious habits and be protective of their kids, which suggested they will undoubtedly suffer and pass their characteristics (and unnerved amygdala) on to individuals later on. On the other hand, early individuals who were too peaceful to even consider evening ponder agonizing over, state, whether or not a lion was nearby or regardless of whether a stream seemed like it would flood their dwelling place, were less inclined to get by and pass on their characteristics. Through ordinary decision, individuals living today are the family members of people whose amygdalae made convincing trepidation responses.

Having a cautious, dread creating amygdala is practically comprehensive among individuals. It isn't surprising, then, that anxiety disorders are the most well- known mental disorder individuals experience, influencing around forty million adults in the United States (Kessler et al. 2005). Considering that the every day hazards in our lives have lessened tremendously since antiquated occasions, you might inquire as to why such countless people are experiencing uneasiness based issues. Sadly, the amygdala is at this point chipping away at the activities it learned in old occasions. It, regardless of everything, trusts us to be potential

prey for various animals or individuals. It anticipates that that the best reaction should hazard is running, fighting, or freezing, and it prepares the body to begin these responses whether or not they're appropriate. Notwithstanding, these dread responses don't fit the twenty-first century conditions that by far most of us live in, and they don't help us in the way in which they once did. For instance, people give off an impression of being leaned to fear snakes, bugs, and statures instead of vehicles, weapons, and plugs, in spite of the way that the last can be more perilous than the past. Also, it similarly creates the impression that a couple of individuals' psyches are progressively helpless against this dread response, whether or not due to inherited characteristics or living through unpleasant experiences.

The Pathways of Anxiety and Fear

Neuroscience incorporates the examination of the improvement, design, and limit of the sensory system, including the mind. To explain the neuroscience of tension, we need to provide you with a compact portrayal of the existence frameworks of the cerebrum, especially of the cortex and the amygdala. Having a grasp of how these huge spaces of the brain work and the way they relate to one another will empower you to get what happens when the cortex or amygdala gets carried away and makes uneasiness. This fundamental data on neuroscience will give you information into how you can modify your psyche to go against anxiety.

THE CORTEX PATHWAY

We'll start with the cortex pathway since when people talk about the mind, they regularly picture the crumpled, faint outer layer of the frontal cortex known as the cerebral cortex. The cortex is brimming with countless humanity's most astounding limits. Regardless, as we'll explain, these limits moreover achieve the cortex being prepared for making a ton of anxiety.

THE CEREBRAL CORTEX

In human, The cortex is greater and has more developed limits than those of different creatures. It's divided into two halves: the left half of the globe and the right side of the equator. It is additionally parceled into different regions, called flaps, that have different limits, for instance, handling vision, hearing, and other material data and collecting it to allow you to see the world. The cortex is the seeing and thinking part about the frontal cortex—the part you're using to scrutinize and comprehend this book.

As well as giving sights, Thusunds, and various perceptions, the cortex in like manner adds significance and recollections to those insights. So, you don't just notice an old individual and hear his voice; rather, you recollect him as your granddad and comprehend the specific significance of the sounds he's making. Additionally, past outfitting you with the ability to comprehend and translate conditions, the cortex licenses you to use rationale and thinking, produce language, use your creative mind, and plan strategies for responding to circumstances.

The cortex can moreover add to changing your responses to undermining conditions, which is key while overseeing nervousness. The cortex is good for evaluating the worth of various responses to the dangers you face. By virtue of the effect of your cortex, you can decide not to really battle your chief assuming you feel you're in danger of being ended or choose not to escape when you hear exploding fireworks. In all honesty, by scrutinizing this book, you're doing the very same thing: viably using your cortex to find different ways to deal with adjust to anxiety.

The cortex pathway to anxiety starts with your sense organs. Your eyes, ears, nose, taste buds, and even your skin are, on the whole, full of information about the world. The entirety of your insight into the world has gotten through your sense organs and been deciphered by different parts of your cortex. At the point when information comes in through your sense organs, it's coordinated to the thalamus, which resembles the Grand Central Station of the cerebrum. The thalamus is a focal transfer station that imparts signs from your eyes, ears, etc. to the cortex. At the point when information comes into the thalamus, it's conveyed to the different lobes to be handled and deciphered. At that point the information goes to different pieces of the cerebrum, including the frontal lobes (behind the temple), where the information is assembled with the goal that you can see and understand the world.

THE FRONTAL LOBES

The front facing projections are one of the main bits of the cortex to comprehend. Found behind the temple and eyes, they're the greatest plan of flaps in the human cerebrum, and they're significantly greater than the front facing projections of

most different animals. The front facing projections get data from the total of various flaps and set up it to allow us to respond to a planned experience of the world. The front facing projections are said to have official limits, suggesting that they are the spot the oversight of numerous frontal cortex structures occurs. The front facing flaps help us with anticipating the eventual outcomes of conditions, plan our exercises, start responses, and utilize input from the world to stop or change our practices. Unfortunately, these stunning cutoff points likewise establish the framework for anxiety.

The cortex pathway is routinely loaded with nervousness in light of the fact that the front facing projections predict and interpret conditions, and assumption and interpretations every now and again lead to tension. For example, assumption can incite another ordinary cortex-based interaction that makes tension: stress. Considering our significantly advanced front facing flaps, individuals can predict future occasions and envision their outcomes—dissimilar to our pets, who seem to rest smoothly without envisioning the upcoming issues. Stress is an outgrowth of assumption for adverse outcomes in a situation. It's a cortex-based cycle that causes considerations that to prompt a great deal of dread and anxiety.

A couple of individuals have a cortex that is magnificent at focusing, taking any situation and envisioning numerous antagonistic outcomes. To be sure, presumably the most imaginative people are moreover now and again the most nervous considering the way that their ingenuity empowers them to bother incredibly alarming thoughts.

An ordinary envisioned concern among guardians who have youngsters who are late (and what kids are not?) is envisioning their kids hurt in a setback, unfit to call for help. This image is startling—and absolutely unessential to envision, be that as it may, a couple of individuals seem to end up on and on anticipating such opposing occasions. If your instance of pushing is sufficient that it interferes with your step by step life, you not really settled to have summed up uneasiness disorder.

Another kind of tension problem, over the top urgent issue, can happen when the front facing projections make fanatical considerations, insights or questions that won't leave, to the point that people go through hours consistently focused on them. Obsessions can to a great extent lead a person to make broad ceremonies that should be done to decrease tension. Consider Jennifer, who examined the sum of the microbes in her home and went through hours cleaning up and cleaning specific domains of her home. By then, later she finished, she'd start by and by considering the fact

that she had questions that drove her to envision that she might have reached something that stained all that she'd cleaned. Such preposterous contemplations may be a direct result of a brokenness in the cingulate cortex, a locale in the front facing projections behind the eyes (Zurowski et al. 2012).

In layout, when we talk about the cortex pathway to tension, we're generally focused on understandings, pictures, and stresses that the cortex makes, or on eager considerations that convey nervousness when no intimidation is free. As referred to, when experts assist people with changing their musings to diminish pressure, they're based on the cortex pathway. Such learned techniques can be exceptionally powerful at diminishing cortex-Initiated nervousness. In any case, as you as of now know, one more neural pathway is moreover connected with the development of tension, regardless, when uneasiness begins in the cortex.

THE AMYGDALA PATHWAY

The resulting pathway incorporates the amygdala. Notwithstanding the way that the cortex pathway to nervousness may be continuously unmistakable or reasonable considering the way that we are consistently aware of the musings it conveys; the amygdala starts the actual experience of uneasiness. Its vital region and affiliations generally through the frontal cortex enable it to control the appearance of chemicals and start zones of the brain that make the actual indications of uneasiness. At this moment, amygdala applies noteworthy and fast effects on the body, and these are vital to understand.

THE AMYGDALA

The amygdala is arranged near the point of convergence of the frontal cortex. As of late communicated, the cerebrum truly has two amygdalae, one in the left half of the globe and one morally justified; nonetheless, it's norm to insinuate the amygdala as one item, so we'll continue with this preparation. The place of your right amygdala can be evaluated by pointing your left index finger at your right eye and your right pointer into your right ear trench. The reason for assembly of the lines from your two fingers is regarding where your right amygdala is found. Since the amygdala is an almond-formed construction, it gets its name from the Greek word for almond. The amygdala is the brimming with a critical number of our passionate reactions, both positive and negative. Exactly when someone ignores your own space or gets in your face, the amygdala conveys the displeasure you feel. On the other hand, when you meet somebody

helps you to remember your grandmother and you experience a warm considered affection for this lady you don't know the first thing about, that is furthermore the amygdala, at the present time a beguiling enthusiastic memory. The amygdala surveys passionate memories; and assuming you get this, your enthusiastic reactions will probably solid great to you.

THE LATERAL NUCLEUS

The amygdala is secluded into a couple of sections; nonetheless, we'll focus chiefly on two that expect central positions in making enthusiastic responses, including fear and nervousness. The horizontal core is the piece of the amygdala that receives moving toward messages from the resources. It persistently channels your encounters and is ready to rock and roll to respond to any indication of hazard. Like a created in caution framework, its obligation is to perceive any danger you see, hear, smell, or feel and a while later grant a risk sign. It gets its data from the thalamus. Honestly, it gets data before the cortex does, and this is basic to remember.

The explanation the horizontal core gets data so speedy is in light of the fact that the amygdala pathway is the more direct course from our resources. The amygdala is wired to respond quickly enough to save your life. Its quick response is possible because of a simple course in cerebrum wiring that grants data to get to the horizontal core of the amygdala clearly (Armony et al. 1995). Right when our eyes, ears, nose, or fingertips get data, the data goes from these receptors to the thalamus, and the thalamus sends this data clearly to the amygdala. At the same time, the thalamus similarly sends the data to the amygdala. At the same time, the thalamus similarly sends the data to the appropriate zones of the cortex for more elevated level handling. In any case, the amygdala gets data before the data can be taken care of by the various flaps in the cortex. This suggests the parallel core of the amygdala can react to safeguard you from danger before your cortex even gets what the danger is.

Information goes from the thalamus to the amygdala, allowing the amygdala to react before you have the chance to use your cortex to think. While this might give off an impression of being odd, assuming you consider your own encounters, you can in all likelihood highlight a couple of times when this has occurred. Have you anytime been in a situation wherein you reacted naturally before you had the chance to know what you were

reacting to?

Consider Melinda, a ten-year-old young lady who was looking for outside gear in the tornado shelter of her home. She walked around a doorway and jumped back in dread. Her reaction was set off by a coat keeping things under control on a coatrack. Her amygdala responded to the condition of the coat, which might have been an interloper and taken her jump a long way from the "intruder" before she even sorted it out what she'd seen. As an improvement based safety effort, the amygdala is wired to react before the cortex can.

The detail-centered cortex saves additional work to deal with data from the thalamus. For Melinda's circumstance, the visual data ought to be shipped off the occipital projection at the back of the head, and starting there it's shipped off the front facing flaps, where the data is incorporated and taught choices arise. That is the explanation Melinda ricocheted back quickly, but recuperated in a second and kept looking for the outside equipment: it stopped briefly for her cortex to give the data that the faint shape was an absolutely innocuous coat.

THE CENTRAL NUCLEUS

The amygdala can accomplish its rapid response because of the uncommon properties of one more core inside it: the focal core. This little yet pivotal pack of neurons has relationship with different extraordinarily incredible constructions in the mind, including the nerve center and the cerebrum stem. This circuit can signal the thoughtful sensory system to start the appearance of chemicals into the circulatory framework, expanded breath, and activate muscles—all in a second.

The close by relationship of the ventral core to parts of the thoughtful sensory system (SNS) outfits the amygdala with a great deal of effect over the body. The SNS is included neurons in the spinal string that interface with about every organ structure in the body, which allows the SNS to affect numerous responses, from understudy expansion to beat. The occupation of the SNS is to make the instinctive reaction, an effect that is changed by the effects of the parasympathetic sensory system (PNS), which licenses us to "rest and digest."

During dread inciting conditions, the parallel core sends messages to the focal core to activate the SNS. All the while, the focal core also authorizes the nerve center. The operational hub controls the appearance of

cortisol and adrenaline, chemicals that set up the body for ensured movement. These chemicals are released from the adrenal organs, arranged on your kidneys. Cortisol builds glucose levels, giving you the solidarity to use your muscles. Adrenaline (furthermore called epinephrine) gives you a blazing tendency that intensifies your resources, builds your heartbeat and breathing and can even safeguard you from feeling torment. These responses begin from the amygdala pathway.

Plainly, the amygdala utilizes a huge load of power concerning beginning a brief moment actual reaction. Somewhat, this is because the amygdala is purposely arranged in a central area of the cerebrum, with brief admittance to data from the resources and a favorable situation to affect bits of the mind that can change fundamental considerable limits quickly. Checking how the amygdala limits are a fundamental piece of the uneasiness riddle.

As ought to be self-evident, one clear distinction between the amygdala and the cortex is that they work on various plans. The amygdala can cause you to circle back to data sooner than your cortex can handle it, orchestrating a genuine response before the cortex has even wrapped up the data so that you could see it. While this is important in specific conditions, the way that we have little authority over the amygdala's fast responses suggests that we experience our dread and uneasiness responses, rather than purposefully controlling them.

The rapid reaction that outcomes from the amygdala pathway are ordinarily called the instinctive reaction. You're doubtlessly familiar with this wonder, which prepares the body to react quickly in a dangerous situation. A significant number of us have experienced this response and can review times we felt an adrenaline flood and reacted in a reckless, brief way to deal with safeguard ourselves from a danger. What quantities of people have been saved money on the turnpike by lightning speedy, natural reactions arising in the amygdala?

The focal anxious of the amygdala is the spot the instinctive response is begun. Checking these speedy responses began by the amygdala pathway can help you with perception and adjust to the actual experience of uneasiness, including the most remarkable tension reaction: a mental episode. People who have a frenzy problem and experience the evil impacts of mental breakdowns believe that it's significant to see that various pieces of a mental breakdown are related to the amygdala's introduction of the instinctive reaction. Pulsating heart, shaking, stomach wretchedness, and hyperventilation are

related to the amygdala's undertakings to set up the body for movement. These signs oftentimes make people figure they might be suffering a heart attack or cardiovascular disappointment or are "going crazy." When people comprehend that the fundamental establishments of a mental episode routinely lie in the amygdala's undertakings to set up the body to respond to an emergency, they're less disposed to be lamented by these concerns (Wilson 2009).

The reactions of acute stress are the most notable dread responses; in any case, the amygdala can similarly make one more response to expect that is less seen: freezing. Believe it or not, we really incline in the direction of the term battle, flight, or freeze response because such a critical number of people state they feel stifled when under unbelievable strain. As peculiar as it shows up, for our forebears the reaction of freezing might have been pretty much as helpful as doing combating or getting away in explicit conditions. Like a bunny that leftover parts unmoving as you walk your canine past her home, the people who freeze now and again find a touch of breathing space in remaining still when compromised.

Exactly when you're experiencing the battle, flight, or freeze response, the amygdala is steering the ship and you're a traveler. That is the explanation, in emergency conditions, you consistently feel as though you're noticing yourself responding rather than deliberately controlling your response. There's an inspiration driving why we don't feel in control at these times, or responsible for our uneasiness: the amygdala isn't just speedier—it similarly has the neurological capacity to annul other mind processes (LeDoux 1996).

There are various relationship from the amygdala to the cortex, allowing the amygdala to solidly affect the cortex's responding on an arrangement of levels, while less associations head out from the cortex to the amygdala (LeDoux and Schiller 2009). Therefore, clearly you can't think when the amygdala takes control. The speculation structures about the cortex are replaced and you're impacted by the amygdala.

Despite the way that you might investigate the worth of this strategy, in specific conditions it's basic. Would it be canny for your psyche to believe that the cortex will explore the make, model, and shade of a vehicle crossing the center line toward you and think about nuances, for instance, the presentation of the driver prior to reacting? Clearly, the limit of the amygdala to cancel the cortex can really save your life. Believe it or not, it apparently at this point has.

Monitoring the amygdala's ability to take over is basic for any person who's engaging with uneasiness. It's an update that the brain is intended to allow the amygdala to clutch control amidst hazard. Furthermore, because of this wiring, it's difficult to use reason-based points of view arising in the more critical levels of the cortex to control amygdala-based uneasiness. You might have recently seen that your nervousness oftentimes doesn't sound great to your cortex, and that your cortex can't just explanation it away.

Furthermore, the amygdala can moreover affect the cortex by causing the appearance of synthetic substances that sway the entire mind, including the cortex (LeDoux and Schiller 2009). These manufactured substances can really change the way in which you think. Along these lines, frameworks for adjusting to amygdala-based tension are essential, regardless of the way that cortex-centered methodologies are generally the more ordinarily presented in treatment.

Considering what you've perused as yet, you ideally comprehend what portions of the cerebrum are related with different kinds of nervousness. You understand that the cortex pathway produces stresses, obsessions, and interpretations that make tension, and you understand that the amygdala fires reactions that make up the battle, flight, or freeze response. Various people find some comfort in knowing where various manifestations are beginning from, that their reactions look good, and that they aren't going insane.

Since you comprehend the pieces of the mind that are related with making uneasiness, you're no doubt captivated by how you can change the way in which these pieces of the cerebrum respond. In order to do in that capacity, you need to make changes in the mind's equipment. The cerebrum is involved billions of related cells that construction circuits that hold your recollections, produce your musings, and start the sum of your exercises. These phones are called neurons, or nerve cells, and they're the fundamental constructions of the mind. They're the clarification that your brain has neuroplasticity: the ability to change itself and its responses. In light of your encounters, the neurons to you are prepared for changing their constructions and instances of reacting. Perceiving how neurons limit will help you with learning processes that will allow you to patch up the circuits in your cerebrum that make nervousness. It will moreover help you with understanding the effects of antianxiety medication on the brain.

Neurons are made from three fundamental parts. The cell body contains the contraption of the cell, including the inherited material that arranges the

construction of the cell. Leaving the cell body are dendrites, which take after parts of a tree. Dendrites are an essential piece of the correspondence system between neurons. They interface with various neurons to receive messages, which head out between neurons to convey messages and produce substances. Dendrites receive messages from the axons of various neurons. The axons don't contact the dendrites; rather, they send their messages by releasing manufactured substances called neural connections into the space between the axon and the dendrite.

The space between an axon and dendrite is known as a neurotransmitter. There, correspondences between neurons occur. Around the finish of the axon, called the axon terminal, minor sacs hold neurotransmitters fully expecting sending mixture messages. A couple of neural connections stimulate the accompanying neuron, and others subdue or quiet it.

Neurotransmitters are called compound specialists since when they cross the synaptic space, they're taking a message to the accompanying neuron. Synapses partner with receptor locales on the dendrites of the accompanying neuron and have an effect like that of setting a key in a lock. We will not go into the specifics, notwithstanding, to lay it out plainly, when a synapses interfaces with the receptor site, it can cause the neuron to react by terminating. Terminating is the place where a positive charge goes from the getting dendrites of a neuron, through the cell body, and right to axons at the far edge. This makes the axon release synapses from its axon terminals, sending the compound message to another neuron, passing the message on.

Neurons work dependent on substance messages among neurons and electrical charges inside neurons. Every sensation you experience, from seeing these words on the page to the traces of flying animals singing in your yard, is ready in your cerebrum by neurons. The sensations you experience, for instance, light waves that enter your eyes or vibrations observable all around that influence your eardrums, get converted into electrical signs inside neurons, and these signs are then granted to various neurons through synapses. By these correspondence frames, the mind collects circuits of neurons that participate to store recollections, make enthusiastic reactions, start perspectives, and produce activities.

At the moment that specialists observed that the messages sent between neurons relied upon synapses sent, beginning with one neuron then onto the next, they began to make sedates that could zero in on this technique. A critical number of the medications most by and large used to treat tension, for instance, Lexapro (escitalopram), Zoloft (sertraline), Effexor (venlafaxine), and Cymbalta (duloxetine), were planned to fabricate the proportion of synapses open in the neural association as a strategy for affecting circuits in explicit zones of the brain.

Why do you have to know how neurons work? On the off chance that you want to patch up the cerebrum, it serves to understanding the mind's hardware and its reason in affiliations formed between neurons. A Canadian therapist named Donald Hebb (1949) proposed a speculation of how neurons make hardware that is wound up being very significant in explaining the strategy. His idea has since been refined into this essential declaration by neuroscientist Carla Shatz: "Neurons that fire together wire together" (Doidge 2007, 63). This message offers clear information into how you can change the wiring in your brain.

Fundamentally, for neurons to create relationship between themselves, one neuron should fire all the while as another neuron is terminating. Right when neurons fire together, a relationship between them is sustained, and in the end an example of hardware makes in which incitation of one neuron causes the other to start as well. More neurons can be related with these neurons in like manner, and in the event that they fire together, soon a whole course of action of related neurons is made. Changing neural hardware incorporates changing the establishment plans in the mind with the objective that new affiliations make among neurons and new circuits structure. Changes in the cerebrum, or learning, can happen as a result of neurons setting up new affiliations and circuitry.

Despite the way that our minds are tweaked from birth to make and figure out themselves, they're amazingly versatile and completely responsive to the particular encounters of each individual. As neuroscientist Joseph LeDoux (2002, 3) explains it, "People don't come preassembled, but are remained together by life." The hardware in your cerebrum is adapted by the specific encounters you've had, and it might be changed on account of your procedure with encounters. For example, relationship between explicit neurons are supported when you use them. A couple of us continue to use our memories of increase tables to figure numerical problems, and those affiliations stay as strong as when we were in school. Nevertheless, a couple of us rely upon adding machines, so we don't regularly use the brain

circuits putting away the duplication tables, thus our memory of these tables degenerates.

The particular circuitry in your brain generates dependent on the experiences you have. Maybe your brain originated to connect ponies with stables, granddads with cigars, the smell of popcorn with baseball, etc. Albeit two individuals may have comparative affiliations, every one of us has particularly framed brain circuits dependent on our own experiences. While one individual may have circuitry that associates cows with cheese and Wisconsin, someone else may have circuitry that associates cows with barns and milking machines.

Neurons make new affiliations and develop new ways in a collection of ways. Circuits can be started by specific cognizant contemplations, like those you have when you're constrained to recall your grandmother. Hardware can be upgraded by changing your conduct, for instance, learning another golf swing. Performing rehearses, like playing the piano or serving a volleyball, can make new circuits make, and regardless, envisioning playing out these practices can cause changes in circuit. The mind stays versatile and fit for making changes generally through life. Assuming you want to change the uneasiness you experience; you need to change the neural affiliations that lead to tension responses. A piece of these affiliations are taken care of in the mind's hardware in the kind of recollections, and recollections are formed in both the cortex and the amygdala.

EMOTIONAL MEMORIES CREATED BY THE AMYGDALA

Emotional recollections are made by the horizontal core in the amygdala through the system of affiliation. These memories start from experiences or occasions that your cortex may review. This is because the memory system in the cortex is completely secluded from that in the amygdala. Believe it or not, research recommends that amygdala-based memory is longer suffering than cortex-based memory (LeDoux 2000). Figuratively speaking, the cortex is extensively almost certain than the amygdala to neglect information or experience trouble recuperating it.

The presence of different memory systems explains why you can experience tension in a situation with no cognizant memory (or perception) of why the situation produces uneasiness. Since your amygdala has an enthusiastic memory of an event doesn't infer that your

cortex reviews a comparable event. Likewise, in the event that your cortex doesn't recall the event, you'll experience inconvenience recollecting that it since we rely upon our cortex memory. This infers that we may, at times, have enthusiastic reactions that puzzle us, especially concerning tension. In this way, you may not comprehend the reason why street crossing points are nervousness impelling, why you avoid sitting with your back to the entrance in a restaurant, or why the smell of tomato plants makes you tense.

The amygdala is good for reacting dependent on its own passionate recollections and shouldn't worry about cortex-based recollections. Research following the pathways in the mind that deal ascend to passionate responses has shown that enthusiastic learning can occur without relationship of the cortex (LeDoux 1996). Here is a model that will assist with delineating this (from Claparede 1951).

A lady was hospitalized in light of Korsakoff's condition, a memory issue every now and again associated with perpetual liquor habit. Her cortex couldn't shape recollections of her experiences, so she couldn't perceive her essential consideration doctor or the clinical center, also the way that she had been in a comparable clinical facility for a significant long time. She didn't have even the remotest clue about the name of the clinical guardian who had pondered her for an impressive time span, and she couldn't remember nuances of a story told to her minutes earlier. But, her amygdala showed the ability to gain enthusiastic experiences without the aide of her cortex.

One day her primary care physician played out a little test (one that wouldn't be moral by the current measures). Right when he associated with shake her hand, he stuck her hand with a pin he'd concealed in his palm. The next day, when the lady saw the expert widen his hand, she promptly pulled back her submit dread. When asked regarding the reason why she would not shake his hand, she couldn't offer an explanation. Also, she uncovered that she had no memory of seeing the expert already. She had no cortex-based memory of an event that would make her dread the trained professional; yet her amygdala had made a passionate memory, and her dread was its proof.

DISCOVERING THE SOURCE OF AMYGDALA-BASED MEMORIES

If you dread a specific article or situation, you may have the choice to audit a contribution with which your amygdala found that dread. Then again, it very well may be difficult to uncover how an amygdala-based fear

made, since your cortex can't recuperate a memory related to that circumstance, regardless of the way that the amygdala clearly does. The way that the cortex can be kept unaware of what's going on is one reason people are consistently puzzled by their passionate reactions.

Here's a manual for diagram what this disarray takes after: Lily saw that she had social fear when she looked into the indications of social fear on a nervousness site. She realized that she felt awkward in gatherings of individuals and that it was hard for her to go to family social occasions, such as Thanksgiving supper or a sister-in-law's baby shower. Exactly when her specialist unveiled to her that this uneasiness was in all likelihood a result of her amygdala, she did not know why her amygdala had developed this enthusiastic response. Notwithstanding, later her expert mentioned that she separate the specific characteristics of the get-togethers that incited nervousness, Lily said that being around of people, even lively family members, was disturbing. She saw that a horde of people was startling to her, especially when they all could check out her all the time.

At the moment that the expert asked regarding whether she could contemplate an encounter that might have shown her amygdala that a horde of people was dangerous, Lily investigated an event in 2nd grade when she was around kids perusing resoundingly from their books so anybody could hear. Right when it was her opportunity to peruse, she encountered issues, and the teacher treated her such that made her vibe humiliated. The cortex-based memory of this involvement with long last got back to Lily, and she comprehended the reason why her amygdala had made a passionate response to endeavor to get her. Considering that memory, her amygdala responded to a horde of people as though they addressed a risk.

Understanding that your amygdala stores enthusiastic recollections that your cortex has no data that can help you with comprehend a part of your passionate reactions. A portion of the time the cortex has a total shortfall of appreciation of the beginnings or explanations behind the passionate reactions made by the amygdala. Be that as it may, you can get to know these systems, so in the accompanying part we'll help you and your cortex become progressively found out with regards to the exercises of the amygdala.

Two pathways can make tension. One pathway dares to all aspects of the detail-centered hardware of the cortex and in the end sends information to the amygdala, which conveys a nervousness response. The other pathway runs from the thalamus to the amygdala. Each pathway can make the amygdala make tension, yet each is moreover worked of individual equipment, and certain pieces of that equipment can be changed. Assuming you perceive how the equipment capacities, you can redo your anxious brain with the objective that you experience less anxiety.

Understanding the Amygdala

Try not to be deceived by the little size of your amygdala. Regardless of the way that the greatest and most muddled piece of the human cerebrum, the cortex, adds to tension according to numerous perspectives, the amygdala expects the most convincing position because, as you learned prior, it's locked in with both the cortex pathway and the amygdala pathway to nervousness. Like the head of an outfit, the amygdala controls a wide scope of reactions in both your frontal cortex and your body. Contingent upon set up responses, it's in like manner completely tricky to what in particular comes to pass for you and responds to your specific encounters.

Right currently, look into the amygdala's exceptional "language" and its impact on your life. In formative terms, the amygdala is an extremely old construction, and the human amygdala is exceptionally similar to the amygdalae found in each and every other animal. Since the human amygdala resembles those in rodents, canines, and even fish, researchers have had the choice to analyze its activities through and through and have taken in a ton regarding how it makes dread and anxiety.

At the moment that you're imagined, your amygdala has coordinated responses that are fit to be utilized in explicit ways. Nevertheless, this old construction isn't fixed; the amygdala is persistently learning and changing ward on your everyday experiences. At the point when you get what we call "the language of the amygdala," you'll have greater authority over your uneasiness responses since you'll understand how to change the part of the mind that is at the actual establishment of fear.

THE AMYGDALA AS A PROTECTOR

To comprehend amygdala-based nervousness, it's important to consider the amygdala your safeguard. Normal choice has given individuals a dread delivering amygdala that has endurance as a principle objective. As you approach your day, the amygdala is vigilant for whatever might show expected damage. While the target of protection is adequate, the amygdala can go

over the edge, making a dread response in conditions that aren't by and large unsafe.

Think about Fran, who will give a discourse. Her heart begins to pound, and she starts to hyperventilate when she remains before the social affair with everyone taking a gander at her. What is her amygdala endeavoring to safeguard her from? It seems like it sees the situation of remaining before a gathering of individuals as unsafe. Fran isn't the only one to experience this kind of response. Studies have shown that dread of public talking is the most widely recognized dread, outflanking apprehension of flying, dread of bugs, dread of statures, and dread of little spaces (Dwyer and Davidson 2012). What could address this typical response? Since the amygdala endeavors to hold us back from being prey to a hunter, formative analysts have prescribed that we may be leaned to deciphering eyes watching us as a perhaps hazardous situation (Ohman 2007). Others have recommended that the risk of excusal by a social occasion of spectators begins from an old dread of being excused by one's clan (Croston 2012), which once implied being abandoned to battle for you and face meandering hunters, essentially the death penalty. In any case, evidently the human amygdala reacts to safeguard us from being in the unprotected situation of being seen by possibly compromising animals, including diverse people.

Fran may not have any familiarity with the formative hidden establishments of her reaction and the amygdala's occupation in it. Her cortex may be uncovering to her that she's restless about being reproached, humiliated, or submitting a mistake, while her amygdala is working according to a logically old perspective. As a matter of fact, the cortex consistently considers purposes behind our practices, which may be exact explanations. Nevertheless, the concern here isn't the precision of the cortex yet its assets. The more Fran harps on cortex-produced explanations for her amygdala-based nervousness, for instance, she's worried that her manager won't be content with this presentation, the more cortex-based uneasiness she'll make, adding to her anxiety. Looking in the cortex for the purposes behind amygdala-based tension takes after looking in your cooler to sort out why your vehicle won't begin. You're not examining the right spot!

Rather, Fran needs to focus on her amygdala's perspective. She wants to see that her amygdala is endeavoring to ensure her. Rather than using her cortex to search for explanations for her tension, she wants to use her cortex to apply her understanding into the language of the amygdala. At first, she really wants to

see that her pulsating heart and quick breathing, which would uphold her assuming she was relied upon to run or battle, don't show that she's truly at risk. These responses are a piece of the amygdala's reaction, and they aren't helpful with respect to public talking. Fran necessities to comprehend this is genuinely not an unsafe situation and that her amygdala is setting off an alarm mistakenly. Whether or not the talk Fran will give is vital, it's impossible that this is the desperate situation that her amygdala is apparently setting up her for.

This highlights the meaning of observing the amygdala's occupation as protector. This is critical in understanding and controlling your own tension responses. Generally speaking, the amygdala's presumption that you ought to be protected from danger is erroneous. Fortunately, you can fix this by retraining your amygdala, and by not giving the amygdala more fuel for the fire by tolerating that a shocking or anxious passionate reaction is a particular indication of hazard. The guarded amygdala reaction is consistently befuddled, and you would rather not let your cortex support the response.

Finally, it's basic to see that basically endeavoring to use your cortex to convince yourself that the situation isn't really unsafe will not generally forestall the amygdala's response. A dynamically convincing philosophy is using breathing techniques and frameworks that retrain the amygdala.

HOW THE AMYGDALA DECIDES WHAT IS DANGEROUS

The human amygdala appears to be inclined to react to certain changes as though they're risky (Ohman and Mineka 2001). Fears of snakes, insects, animals, heights, anger, and disease appear to be naturally wired into the amygdala, since people learn them with next to no provoking. For example, barely does any kid have a dread of vehicles, yet many dread bugs. Regardless of the way that vehicles address a considerably more genuine danger to youngsters than bugs, the dread of bugs is apparently planned into the amygdala with the ultimate objective that kids develop this dread with no issue. This is beyond question the result of thousands of extended lengths of progression where a dread of bugs contributed here and there or one more to endurance. Notwithstanding, even sensations of dread that are tweaked into the amygdala can be changed. Assuming it demonstrated unfit to change, it's far-fetched that such a critical number of us would live with sharp-toothed creatures like felines or canines and treat them as a piece of our families.

Then once more, various things or conditions aren't typically dreaded by the amygdala. Rather, the amygdala sorts out some way to fear them due to life experiences. The amygdala is ceaselessly learning subject to encounter, and later certain critical experiences, it makes cerebrum circuits that make people dread a once in the past unfeared object. For example, a youngster doesn't ordinarily fear a fire and ought to be advised not to get in touch with it. Regardless, later a kid is singed by, say, a birthday light, the kid's amygdala sorts out some way to fear by seeing fire. Similarly, the amygdala quickly adds distinctive blasting items to its summary of dangerous things to avoid, so the youngster may moreover fear lighters, sparklers, and outdoors fires. The amygdala holds suffering memories that recognize the article and relative things as hazardous. This is an amazingly noteworthy and flexible limit, since it considers the development of specific neural equipment that helps people with sidestepping the specific dangers that occur in their lives. This has kept the amygdala accommodating and basically unaltered for some years.

At the moment that we reveal the two pathways to tension to people, they often ask concerning whether they might have procured a sensitive amygdala. Genetic characteristics can affect the amygdala and as such your generally common enthusiastic reactions. For example, kids who have a more modest left amygdala will overall have more tension inconveniences than different kids (Milham et al. 2005). The inspiring news is, every amygdala is good for learning and changing, and in later parts you'll sort out some way to set up your amygdala to respond in an unforeseen way.

As inspected already, the amygdala structures recollections, yet not in the way wherein people regularly think about memories. In view of your experiences, your amygdala makes passionate memories—both positive and negative—that you don't actually have a knowledge of. Positive passionate recollections, for instance, the relationship of the smell of aroma with feelings of friendship for your associate, ordinarily don't bring a ton of hardship. Consequently, we'll base on bad enthusiastic recollections, especially those that achieve dread and uneasiness, because these recollections can cause a ton of amygdala-based anxiety.

As indicated partially 1, the parallel core of your amygdala gains passionate experiences reliant upon your experiences, and these memories can lead you to respond to explicit things or conditions like they're dangerous. In light of these recollections, you're mindful of an opinion of burden, dread, or fear. Regardless, you don't comprehend that this tendency is a direct result of a passionate memory considering the way that the memory isn't taken care of as an image or verbal information. It isn't similar to for an old photo diagram or film in your cerebrum, as cortex-based recollections can be.

Rather, you experience an amygdala-based memory clearly, as a passionate state. You essentially begin feeling a specific inclination. Assuming it so happens that this inclination is uneasiness, it's everything except hard to expect that having a ghastly or nervous inclination is a careful impression of the danger of a circumstance on the off chance that you don't comprehend the language of the amygdala. Contemplate Sam, who was in an auto crash that genuinely hurt his better half, who was driving. Straight up to now, when he rides in the front seat of a vehicle, Sam has nervousness—a squeezing feeling of danger that seems to result from the force situation in his condition. Sam doesn't experience a memory of the setback or consider the accident each time he experiences this amygdala-based uneasiness. Regardless, at whatever point he pushes toward the front seat, he has a strong tendency that he should avoid the situation, and he ends up being incredibly off-kilter and essentially panicky whenever he endeavors to ride with another driver. Assuming he endeavors to verbalize his opinions, he says it seems like something horrendous will happen on the off chance that he rides in the front seat. He's logically open to driving himself, and for a significant long time he's kept away from being a voyager. Since his significantly felt enthusiastic reaction is so real and enduring, he doesn't consider whether he should address it. He would never depict it as a memory outlined by his amygdala, and he doesn't guess that he ought to change it or even comprehend that he can.

THE FIGHT, FLIGHT, OR FREEZE RESPONSE

As referred to previously, the amygdala's central region in the cerebrum places it in a great circumstance to affect various bits of the brain that can change major considerable limits in a modest quantity of a second. Exactly when danger is recognized, the amygdala can impact different astoundingly amazing designs in the cerebrum, including the mind stem excitement structures, the nerve center, the hippocampus, and the core accumbens. These quick affiliations grant the amygdala to, instantly, start motor (advancement) structures, stimulate the insightful sensory system, increment levels of neurotransmitters, and release chemicals like adrenaline and

cortisol into the circulatory framework. This establishment makes a course of changes in the body: beat expands, the circulation system is created some distance from the stomach related plot to the uttermost places, muscles tense, and the body is animated and ready for action. Considering these physiological changes, you might feel shuddering, a thumping heart, and stomach trouble.

These movements are a piece of the battle, flight, or freeze response, and as noted ahead of time, the focal core is the piece of the amygdala where the battle, flight, or freeze response is begun. Exactly when this reaction is required, we consider it a lifesaving event. Regardless, assuming the focal core overcompensates, it can set off an all out mental episode when no genuine reason behind dread exists. At the point when it begins a mental episode, the focal core of the amygdala is in control and the cortex has close to no effect. A couple of individuals respond powerfully when they are frightened, some break the circumstance, and others are immobilized. In the event that you're throwing a tantrum of nervousness and people endeavor to outfit you with lucid motivations behind why you shouldn't freeze, they're essentially speaking with a cortex that is disconnected. Frameworks that emphasis on the amygdala, for instance actual development or breathing, will be progressively dynamic however.

Monitoring the amygdala's ability to accept accountability is basic for any person who battles with uneasiness. It fills in as an update that everyone's mind is intended to allow the amygdala to keep up with control amidst hazard. Multitudinous presences (of individuals and various animals) have been saved by the amygdala's ability to quickly order significant reactions in dangerous conditions. Models remember pounding for the brakes in busy time gridlock, avoiding when a foul ball is voyaged your course, or leaving the room when the veins in your administrator's neck are enlarging. These conditions are events when your amygdala is attempting to save you from a danger. Notwithstanding, as we referred to, a portion of the time the benevolent amygdala is itself the disorder.

Now, you've taken in a ton regarding how the amygdala makes tension. You comprehend that one of the essential components of the amygdala is to get you. You similarly understand that it can recognize specific things or conditions as hazardous, by and large considering a learning experience. You found that the amygdala gains notice of experiences that you may not know about, but which you experience as feelings. Finally, you understand that the amygdala has

a fast response system that can take over both your frontal cortex and your body when it feels that you're at significant danger. This raises the issue of how we can rehearse authority over the amygdala. To do in that capacity, we need to pass on new information to this little yet noteworthy piece of the brain, and the best way achieve this is by using the amygdala's own language.

We use "language" here to depict the technique for correspondence between the amygdala and the rest of the world. This particular language isn't words, yet it is sentiments. With respect to uneasiness, the language of the amygdala has a really slender focus on hazard and prosperity. It relies upon comprehension, and it's a language of lively movement and response. Right when you comprehend the points of interest of this language, your experiences with amygdala-based uneasiness will look good, and you'll moreover have the choice to convey new information to your amygdala in order to set it up to respond in a surprising way.

As discussed already, a focal law principal the neural circuits in the cerebrum is "neurons that fire together wire together" (Doidge 2007, 63). The amygdala's language relies upon making relationship between neurons. With respect to amygdala-based uneasiness, relationship between neurons are made when material data about a thing or situation is being ready by neurons in the equal center of the amygdala while something compromising ends up invigorating the amygdala. In any compromising circumstance, the amygdala is endeavoring to recognize any sight, sound, or other substantial information identified with the danger. Along these lines, affiliation is a fundamental piece of the language of the amygdala.

Clinicians have pondered affiliation based learning, commonly called old style molding, for longer than a century, but in the new many years have they seen that a couple of sorts of this learning occur in the amygdala. There have been various revelations from neuroscientist Joseph LeDoux (1996) and his group, who are investigating the neurological reason of amygdala-based uneasiness. The amygdala really takes a look at the substantial pieces of your life and responds in obvious habits when material information is related with positive or negative events happening all the while. Right when sensations, things, or conditions have been connected with a negative event, memories are taken care of by the level center in circuits that are

wired to convey a negative feeling.

Envision an individual being stood up to by a canine. The sights and hints of the canine are ready through the thalamus and gave off clearly to the sidelong center of the amygdala, which doesn't naturally roll out an improvement in neural equipment that will cause uneasiness. Neurons in the equal center change so that dread is discovered just assuming tangible data about the canine is being ready in the sidelong core going before or all the while as the occasion of a negative experience, for instance, being compromised or chomped by the canine. Thusly, in the event that the canine carries on in an amicable or impartial manner, the horizontal core won't make a negative enthusiastic memory about the dog.

For any situation, when a horrifying or negative experience like a canine nibble occurs, the neurons sending the tangible data about the chomp make intense passionate excitation in the parallel core. Assuming this excitation is going on at about a comparative time that the horizontal core is tolerating tactile information about the canine, the parallel core changes neural hardware to respond adversely to canines or similar animals later on. In investigations on rodents, scientists have truly had the choice to see that affiliation's construction in the amygdala when such pairings are capable (Quirk, Repa, and LeDoux 1995).

An item or circumstance itself need not be hurtful or compromising for fear or anxiety to be related with it. Any article, even a teddy bear, can come to cause anxiety through association-based learning. For a relationship to grow, all that is required is that the object be competent at about a similar time that some stirring or compromising occasion is enacting the lateral nucleus. Keep in mind, neurons become associated when they're firing simultaneously. The association-based language of the amygdala is the thing that makes a considerable lot of the emotional responses you experience; amygdala-based anxiety is just a single model. On account of anxiety, the horizontal core associate's tangible data from a circumstance with the feeling of fear. After this association has been made, you'll feel on edge at whatever point the amygdala perceives comparative tangible information. The sights, sounds, or scents related with the negative occasion become fit for actuating the amygdala's alert framework. The term trigger alludes to anything—an occasion, object, sound, smell, etc. that actuates the amygdala's alarm framework because of association based learning. In the model above, dogs become a trigger for anxiety. Triggers are a significant part of the language of the amygdala.

It may give off an impression of being astonishing that any item can transform into a trigger assuming it's dealt with when the amygdala is in a sanctioned state. Regardless, amygdala-based uneasiness is a direct result of affiliations, not rationale, so triggers don't have to seem OK. Here is a model that addresses how affiliation, not conditions and sensible outcomes, oversees amygdala-based tension: Josefina was acquainting a teddy hold on for her grandson, who was running happily toward her. By then he out of the blue fell and split his lip open on the carport. By and by he experiences amygdala-based uneasiness whenever he sees a teddy bear. Since the magnificently harmless teddy bear was connected with the aggravation of the injury, the teddy bear transformed into a trigger, provoking a dread of teddy bears.

The amygdala's reaction might go from commonly delicate to incredibly strong, dependent upon the experience. For instance, you might have a smooth severe dislike of a particular kind of sustenance that was connected with a negative experience, for example, a serving of blended greens that you ate during a disagreeable family picnic. On the other hand, assuming you once ate pancakes when you had an infection that later made you upchuck, you might observe that, even a long time afterward, essentially the smell of hotcakes makes you nauseous.

Before you get the likelihood that you might be in an optimal circumstance without your amygdala, remember that its responsibility is to guarantee you.

Additionally, it produces good sentiments in view of affiliation based learning. For example, in the event that your companion gives you an extra as a gift, you'll experience opinions of warmth and love for them. A short time later, when you see the gems, the affiliation outlined between the accessory and the sensation of reverence will make you experience warm and affection feelings again. Had the extra not been coordinated with a companion or relative, it would basically be one more piece of embellishments. Various positive passionate reactions are conveyed by the amygdala, so you wouldn't want to discard it.

Truth be told, in the event that two people have had different experiences, they can have absolutely different reactions to a comparative article, because of the language of the amygdala. Catherine has friendly affections for daddy longleg bugs, since she as frequently as conceivable experienced them while picking her favored red raspberries in her grandmother's nursery. She has been known to delicately get daddy longlegs and eliminate them from her home, to the repugnance of her

companion Elizabeth, whose amygdala reacts to daddy longlegs as though they're horrible.

EXERCISE: IDENTIFYING AMYGDALA EMOTIONS IN YOUR LIFE

Would you be able to recognize innocuous circumstances or items that inspire amygdala-based anxiety because of the association-based language of your amygdala? Have you at any point been confused by your response to a person or thing you had no rhyme or reason to fear? Additionally, consider whether you've anytime experienced frightening good sentiments considering someone or something. These enthusiastic responses could be an impression of the language of the amygdala. On an alternate piece of paper, list occurrences of both positive and negative reactions. Remember, the things you list for either characterization need not be intrinsically positive or negative things. For example, you might have a negative enthusiastic reaction to the aroma of lilacs and a good passionate reaction to lightning storms.

THE AMYGDALA'S REACTIONS AREN'T LOGICAL

As ought to be self-evident, amygdala-based sentiments aren't normal. They're established on affiliations, not rationale. Contemplate Beth, who was assaulted while a specific Rolling Stones song was playing. Later the trap, whenever Beth heard the tune, she felt remarkable tension. Unmistakably, the Rolling Stones tune didn't have anything to do with the attack; it was possibly chance that it was playing when the assault occurred. Regardless,

Beth's amygdala responded to the connection between the song and the assault, an inconceivably regrettable event. Hence, the amygdala changes a fair-minded article or circumstance into something that makes a passionate reaction. To be progressively correct, the actual thing isn't changed; rather, it's dealt with in another course by the amygdala.

Individuals experience the affiliation the amygdala makes between an item and dread, yet they may not see or comprehend the affiliation. They might feel a convincing enthusiastic reaction to a thing without understanding that a neural affiliation has been made or under-standing why the passionate reaction is occurring. This shortfall of care is absolutely commonplace and connects with a wide scope of neural limits. For example, you don't should be purposefully aware of the neural circuits that license you to examine this book, to sit up, or to unwind. Thank sky! That kind of care would be devastating.

However, for people who have tension, having a comprehension of the amygdala's colossal occupation in making dread affiliations is valuable. It grants you to stop looking for shrewd explanations and start sorting out some way to use the language of the amygdala. We'll utilize Don, a Vietnam veteran with post-awful pressure issue (PTSD) for example of how having a grasp of the language of the amygdala can be helpful. Wear used to have alarm assaults, and afterward didn't have one for quite a while. Suddenly, he started throwing a tantrum of tension each day for no clear clarification. Exactly when encouraged to explore the situation, Don comprehended that his frenzy was solidly associated with showering. Following several significant length of watching his tension work as he showered, Don comprehended that his better half had changed to a comparative brand of cleaning agent that he'd used in Vietnam. The smell of the cleanser was inciting an amygdala response and making alarm assaults. In the language of the amygdala, the cleanser was a trigger identified with the war.

Perceiving that the cleanser was the clarification behind his mental episodes was an assistance for Don. Knowing the language of the amygdala gave him another agreement that assisted him with seeing that he wasn't going crazy and that his PTSD wasn't starting to accept command over his life again, something he was particularly stressed over. For Don's circumstance, understanding the language of the amygdala was helpful, in spite of the way that it didn't end his uneasiness. He actually felt nervous at whatever point he smelled the chemical, notwithstanding understanding that the cleaning agent wasn't hazardous; regardless, he could stop his morning alarm assaults by changing to a substitute brand of cleanser.

For Don, avoiding that brand of cleanser had no costs. Notwithstanding, a couple of times the trigger is something progressively irksome, or unimaginable, to avoid. Consider a jack of all trades who has a dread of unpleasant little creatures (which have a technique for stowing away under sinks), or an office manager who works on the 20th floor and has alarm assaults in lifts. In these cases, decreasing or taking out the dread or mental episodes requires retraining the amygdala. It is possible that you don't know where a particular passionate reaction started from. Fortunately, it isn't critical to know the principal justification for amygdala-based tension to change the passionate hardware. At the point when you notice that a specific trigger is connected with an uneasiness response, you can figure out how to change the equipment related with that trigger, whether or not you don't have even the remotest clue about the primary justification behind the passionate memory.

Numerous people acknowledge that the results of tension problem, for instance, frenzy, stress, and avoiding of explicit things or conditions, should be decreased by solid conflict. Benevolent family members and associates, and, sometimes, even people doing combating with tension, regularly figure rationale and reason should change the way in which the anxious individual reacts. Regardless, clearly, the amygdala isn't reasonable. For instance, assuming a small kid fears canines directly following being bit by one, you will not go anyplace by saying, "Don't worry about my canine Buddy. He's never chomped anyone. He's essentially innocuous." Once you have a grasp of the language of the amygdala, it's sensible why rationale based mediations miss the mark. As you'll see later in the book, various cortex-based nervousness secondary effects do respond to predictable conflicts, yet with regards to amygdala-based uneasiness, there's simply a solitary sure course for the amygdala to learn: understanding.

The amygdala's reliance on experience for learning explains why significant length of talk treatment or managing different self improvement guides may not assist with tension: they may not be zeroing in on the amygdala. Assuming that you really want the amygdala to change its response to a thing (for example, a mouse) or a situation, (similar to an uproarious gathering), the amygdala needs association in the article or situation for new comprehension to occur. Experience is best when the singular interfaces straightforwardly with the article or situation, but watching another person has moreover been seemed to impact the amygdala (Olsson, Nearing, and Phelps 2007). You can sway the amygdala for an extensive timeframe, yet on the off chance that you're endeavoring to change amygdala-based tension, that methodology will not be just about as amazing as two or three snapshots of direct experience will be.

Thusly, to change your amygdala's dread response to, say, a mouse, you ought to be inside seeing a mouse to start the memory circuits related to mice. At precisely that point, new affiliations can be made. Since the amygdala learns dependent on affiliations or pairings, it should encounter a change in these pairings for the hardware to change. As anybody would expect, when your mouse-memory circuits are initiated, you will feel some anxiety.

Tragically, people normally endeavor to avoid such experiences, and this avoidance holds the amygdala back from molding new associations. Returning to the instance of the mouse, you might even endeavor to avoid thinking about mice, considering the way that essentially the possibility of a

mouse can make the amygdala react, beginning an uneasiness response. The amygdala will overall defend learned passionate reactions by avoiding any show to the trigger, which lessens the likelihood of changing that enthusiastic equipment. Being an authoritative survivalist, the amygdala is purposefully careful, and its default setting is to figure out responses that decay first experience with triggers. Regardless, again, amygdala-based nervousness responses won't change assuming the amygdala is viable in staying away from triggers.

At the moment that you manage the likelihood that you need to establish the amygdala's circuits to deliver new affiliations, you've taken in a huge exercise. We like the succinct articulation "enact to create" as shorthand for this need, which is perhaps the most difficult exercise in the language of the amygdala. It's troublesome considering the way that it incorporates enduring the experience of uneasiness as fundamental for new comprehension to occur. By partaking in experiences that start the amygdala's memory of a specific article or situation, you convey to the amygdala in its own language and put it in the best circumstance for new circuits to outline and new comprehension to happen.

SYNOPSIS

Right now, you have sorted out how the amygdala makes uneasiness on account of the affiliations it experiences. You've found that one of the central components of the amygdala is to guarantee you, and that the amygdala makes memories that you may not as yet know about experience rather as passionate reactions. The amygdala has a prompt response system that can take over both your mind and your body when it feels you're at risk. In any case, the amygdala can acquire from its experiences, and you can use the amygdala's own language of relationship to make new affiliations. You'll later sort out some way to modify the amygdala, so it responds in a calm manner.

Regardless of the way that the amygdala pathway is pivotal in its ability to start an arrangement of actual reactions in a brief moment, uneasiness can likewise have its beginning in the cortex pathway. The cortex works in something else altogether in contrast with the amygdala; in any case, its responses and hardware can affect the amygdala to convey tension. Through this strategy, the cortex can make inconsequential uneasiness and moreover escalate nervousness that starts in the amygdala. At the point when you perceive how your cortex

starts or adds to nervousness, you can see the opportunities for either blocking or modifying cortex reactions to diminish your anxiety.

CAUSES OF ANXIETY IN THE CORTEX

The cortex can cause uneasiness in two general habits. The first incorporates how the cortex structures tangible data, for instance, sights and sounds. As discussed, the thalamus guides material information to the cortex, similarly with respect to the amygdala. As the cortex shapes this information, it can unravel perfectly safe sensations as undermining. It by then conveys something explicit along to the amygdala that can convey tension. At the present time, cortex turns a genuinely fair experience that wouldn't ordinarily impel the amygdala into a danger, causing the amygdala to react by making a nervousness reaction.

Here's a model: An auxiliary school senior who had applied to a couple of colleges investigated the mail and saw an envelope from one of the colleges he'd applied to. Imagining that it contained an excusal letter, he had several amazingly anxious minutes prior to opening the envelope. As it ended up, he'd been acknowledged and had even been conceded a grant. In light of everything, his cortex began a tension response by interpreting seeing the envelope to such an extent that made upsetting contemplations, and these considerations authorized his amygdala. This kind of cortex-put together uneasiness depends with respect to the cortex's interpretation of the tactile data it gets.

The second expansive way the cortex can begin a tension response occurs without the incorporation of a specific external sensations. For example, when pushes or alarming contemplations are made in the cortex, this can start the amygdala to convey a nervousness response regardless of the way that the individual hasn't seen, heard, or felt anything that's hazardous in any way. A model would be gatekeepers of an infant youngster who pass on their child with a sitter to go out for dinner and out of the blue begin to have stresses over their kid's security. Notwithstanding the way that the kid is completely ensured, the gatekeepers imagine that he's in a difficult situation or being excused by the sitter. Musings like these can start the amygdala in spite of the way that there's no material information exhibiting that the kid is at genuine risk.

COGNITIVE FUSION

Before we review these two general habits by which the cortex makes nervousness, we really want to address a method that can occur in both: scholarly blend, or taking confidence in the reality of minor considerations. It's maybe the

most concerning issue made in the cortex, which can convey an unyielding conviction that contemplations and sentiments should be treated as though they reflect an outrageous reality that can't be tended to. Both the optional school senior and the focused on gatekeepers in the models above may have capitulated to mental blend by taking their negative contemplations too genuinely.

Mistaking a thought for the fact of the matter is outstandingly captivating. On account of the cortex's penchant to trust, it trusts every thought, feeling, or actual sensation is genuine. In actuality, the cortex is incredibly disposed to misinterpretations and errors. It's totally expected to have erroneous, preposterous, or nonsensical contemplations, or to experience sentiments that don't look good. When in doubt, you want not take every thought or feeling you have truly. You can allow various contemplations and sentiments to simply do without excessive thought or examination. We will later inspect mental blend exhaustively, help you with looking over whether you're leaned to scholarly mix, and give strategies to help you with stopping this.

ANXIETY THAT ARISES INDEPENDENTLY FROM SENSORY INFORMATION

Presently we'll explore the different ways the cortex can begin tension. In the first place, we'll consider the kind of nervousness that beginnings as musings made by the cortex, without any information from your resources. There are truly two subcategories of this method—thought-based and symbolism based—and each conventionally arises in a substitute portion of the mind of the cortex, with thought-based tension starting from the left half of the equator and imagery based uneasiness beginning from the right. Taking everything into account; these two kinds of cortex-based uneasiness aren't on a very basic level disconnected. Honestly, they consistently happen together.

LEFT HEMISPHERE BASED ANXIETY

Troubling considerations will undoubtedly start in the left 50% of the cortex, which is the dominating side of the side of the equator for language in a great many people. Legitimate thinking, which is conveyed in the left 50% of the cerebrum, underlies both pressure and verbal rumination (Engels et al. 2007). Stress is the way toward envisioning adverse outcomes for a circumstance. Rumination is a way of thinking that incorporates needlessly thinking about issues, associations, or possible conflicts. In rumination, there's a genuine focus on the subtleties and

expected causes or effects of conditions (Nolen-Hoeksema 2000). Despite the way that people might feel that things like pressure or rumination will provoke a reply, what truly happens is a building up of the equipment in the cortex that produces nervousness. In like manner, rumination has been believed to provoke distress (Nolen-Hoeksema 2000). Whatever you commit a ton of time to considering exhaustively will undoubtedly be built up in your cortex. The circuits in the brain work on the standard of "endurance of the most active" (Schwartz and Begley 2003, 17), and whatever hardware you use drearily is presumably going to be adequately started later on. This suggests rather than inciting game plans, the methodology of stress and rumination make significant dejections in your thinking processes that make you, as a general rule, focus on these concerns in your left half of the side of the equator. At times, people become stirred up in separating circumstances on various occasions, making an experience called anxious dread (Engels et al. 2007). As these enduring, upsetting considerations are polished over and over in the mind, they become continuously difficult to pardon. This sort of thinking is especially normal among people with summed up uneasiness issue and fanatical habitual disorder.

RIGHT HEMISPHERE–BASED ANXIETY

The human ability to imagine conditions exhaustively begins from the right 50% of the cortex, which takes a gander at the world uniquely in contrast to the informative, verbal, left half of the equator. The advantaged hemi-circle is nonverbal and structures things in progressively widely inclusive, facilitated ways. It causes us see plans, see faces, and perceive and express sentiments. It in like manner gives us visual pictures, creative mind, dreams, and sense. Because of these cutoff points, it can add to tension, reliant upon inventive psyche and perception.

At the moment that you apparently imagine something disturbing, you use the right half of the cortex to do thusly. Exactly when you hear the fundamental tone of allegations in your innovative psyche, your right half of the side of the equator is incorporated. On the off chance that you're particularly satisfactory at using your innovative psyche, you can expect your amygdala to respond. The amygdala can end up being significantly actuated when the right 50% of the half of the globe makes startling pictures.

Research recommends that the right half of the side of the equator is insistently associated with nervousness appearances (Keller et al. 2000). In all honesty, it's

more vehemently related than the left 50% of the side of the equator with the kind of uneasiness wherein a singular feels strong energy and genuine dread (Engels et al. 2007). For example, people with alarm assaults will undoubtedly have right 50% of the side of the equator based nervousness (Nitschke, Heller, and Miller 2000). Along these lines, when you're feeling strong, animating nervousness, rather than unfortunate or stress-based uneasiness, the right half of your cortex will undoubtedly be incited. Watchfulness, an overall state of availability where the whole condition is inspected for indications of danger, is also arranged in the right half of the side of the equator (Warm, Matthews, and Parasuraman 2009).

By and by we'll go to the following sort of cortex-based nervousness portrayed close to the beginning of the segment: uneasiness that rises up out of the cortex's interpretations of fair tangible data. Incidentally, you may be in a situation that is faultlessly shielded, yet your cortex responds to tactile data like it's dangerous or disturbing. Information beginning from your capacities through the thalamus is given importance by the way that the circuits in the cortex technique and decipher that information. Could we return to the instance of the optional school understudy who thought he was being excused by a school anyway was really being offered a grant. His cortex had translated an envelope as a cause of disturbing news and changed it into a very surprising item.

The front facing projections of the human cortex have an all around created capacity to inspect future events and imagine their outcomes. This is consistently exceptionally obliging, with the cortex conveying translations that license us to respond well to an assortment of conditions. Regardless, messes start when the cortex at least a few times reacts in habits that produce uneasiness. Whether or not in light of specific learning experiences, explicit physiological methodology, or, generally a significant part of the time, a mix of both, the hardware in the cortex can respond in habits that advance pressure, skepticism, and other negative interpretive procedures.

If your cortex translates an immaculately shielded situation as undermining, you'll feel nervousness. Contemplate Damon, who strolls his canine in his area. He sees a fire motor going toward his home with its lights on and cautions impacting and unravels this to infer that his house is burning. As needs be, he starts to feel colossal tension. The justification for his tension is that his cortex comprehends the significance of a fire motor, not just the fire motor as an item: an accident or wellbeing related emergency that doesn't has anything to do

with a fire or Damon's house isn't thought of. Rather than pondering these other options, Damon imagines that his house is on fire. As needs be, his passed on side of the mind gets the chance to work considering the habits where a discharge might have started, figuring, *I might have left the oven on or The wiring is so old. Perhaps a short gotten a fire going.* Meanwhile, his right 50% of the cerebrum is making photos of his kitchen drenched ablaze. His amygdala is most likely going to react to such contemplations, and likewise, Damon might flood home in a frenzy, regardless of the way that there's no certified danger to his home. His interpretation is the wellspring of his anxiety.

ANTICIPATION: THE GIFT OF THE HUMAN CORTEX

Since the human cortex can predict future events and imagine their results, we experience assumption, which is both a gift and a revile. Expectation, which implies assumptions regarding what will occur, relies upon the cortex's ability to begin preparing for a future event by considering or envisioning it. It happens chiefly in the prefrontal cortex (which lies behind the sanctuary) on the left, progressively verbal side. The left prefrontal cortex is the piece of the frontal cortex where we plan and execute exercises, so it's not shocking that assumption arises here, as it's connected to getting ready to act some way or another or another. We can imagine in good habits and have a stimulated and invigorated outlook on a best in class event. Regardless, we can similarly predict in bad ways, expecting and imagining negative or even unsafe events. This can incite a ton of misery.

The assumption for negative conditions creates compromising considerations that can essentially assemble uneasiness. To be sure, the experience of assumption is consistently more disturbing than the predicted event itself! When in doubt, the musings people have about a best in class situation, for instance, an expected a showdown, a test, or a task that should be done, are significantly more awful than the certifiable situation winds up being.

As ought to be self-evident, the cortex's ability to use language, produce pictures, and imagine the future licenses it to begin a nervousness response in the amygdala regardless, when no reason behind tension exists. People when in doubt feel that its easier to see the cortex's occupation in making tension than the amygdala's work. This is because we're logically prepared to watch and comprehend the language of musings delivered in the cortex. A couple of bits of the cortex are more vigorously impacted by us than the amygdala is,

and we're progressively prepared to frustrate and change cortex-made musings. In light of everything; we don't plan to suggest that controlling the cortex is straightforward. Your cortex has developed explicit instances of responding, and whenever it has developed these affinities, it will in general be hard to ruin and change them.

THE FINAL STEP IN THE CORTEX PATHWAY TO ANXIETY: THE AMYGDALA

Conversation of the cortex pathway isn't done until we address the occupation of the last part in the pathway: the amygdala. Isolated, the cortex can't make a nervousness response; the amygdala and various pieces of the mind are relied upon to accomplish that. In all honesty, people without a functioning amygdala, whether or not due to stroke, illness, or injury, don't experience dread in the way in which by far most of individuals do.

Consider the case of a lady whose amygdalae were both destroyed by an uncommon condition, Urbach-Wiethe sickness (Feinstein et al. 2011). Her story offers a gander at what life looks like without the amygdala's dread response. She can be introduced to bugs or snakes or watch disturbing scenes from violence films without experiencing dread. Significantly more astoundingly, over the range of her day to day existence, she was held up at gunpoint and, moreover, was almost killed during an assault, but experienced no dread in one or the other situation. Honestly, she's been the setback of a grouping of infringement, probably because she doesn't have the readiness that would rise out of a functioning amygdala. Her experiences address that the amygdala is the wellspring of the dread response. Notwithstanding what musings, pictures, or wants start in the cortex, countless the enthusiastic and physiological pieces of nervousness result exactly when the cortex starts the amygdala.

The amygdala responds to information passed on from the cortex. Honestly, the amygdala might respond to what we imagine comparatively that it responds to what exactly's truly happening. Information subject to considerations of potential danger dares to all aspects of undefined pathways from information related with certified observations and interpretations. As discussed previously, the amygdala quickly frames information it gets from the resources through the thalamus. Later a deferment during which the cortex structures and interprets the information, the amygdala similarly gets data from the cortex. Neuroscientists don't yet realize exactly how the amygdala perceives whether the information it gets from the cortex is significant, or reliant upon an overactive imagination.

We should investigate two occasions of how the amygdala might respond to contemplations made in the cortex, to check out how the amygdala's reliance on the cortex can be either useful or tricky. In the principle model, Charlotte is at home one night when she hears the natural sound of someone returning in the doorway. She hears this uproar reliably when her better half gets back home, so her amygdala doesn't respond to the sound as an indication of danger. Regardless, Charlotte knows in her cortex that her life partner is away on a fishing trip and that no one should be returning in the entrance at the present time. Her cortex produces musings of danger and an image of a more peculiar entering her home. These contemplations in Charlotte's cortex sway her amygdala to begin the battle, flight, or freeze response. Charlotte's heart starts thumping and she stops what she's doing. She becomes hyper careful and bases on getting herself to wellbeing. Assuming that there is a gatecrasher, these reactions could save her life.

Charlotte's amygdala isn't responding to the entryway. It's responding to Charlotte's contemplations that there may be an outsider in the house. Responding to information from the cortex allows the amygdala to get ready for risks it doesn't see. The amygdala relies upon the cortex to give it additional information. However, a portion of the time the amygdala's reliance on the cortex prompts pointless uneasiness, as in the accompanying model.

Right now, she is without a doubt alone at home while her better half is away. She hears nothing odd, yet she feels awkward when she hits the hay. As she lies in bed, checking out the quiet evening, she imagines that someone is breaking into the house. She imagines an interloper walking around inside the house with a weapon, and her amygdala responds to these photos in her cortex. In spite of the way that there's no quick verification that she's in any hazard, her amygdala responds to the development in her cortex by beginning the battle, flight, or freeze reaction. Out of the blue, Charlotte feels a terrible sensation of dread. Her breathing gets shallow and she accepts she should conceal or search for help, notwithstanding the way that she comprehends that there's no strong verification of peril.

Charlotte's amygdala is responding to the contemplations in her cortex like they reflect genuine hazard, and it makes an unquestionable dread response. As ought to be clear from these two models, what you consider and revolve around in the cortex can impact your level of uneasiness. From the perspective of the amygdala, considerations in the cortex might require a response, whether or not simply the amygdala doesn't recognize hazard from the tangible data it got. In reacting to the cortex's information, the amygdala might begin the battle, flight, or freeze reaction. Likewise, when the amygdala gets included, you begin to experience the actual sensations related with anxiety.

Luckily, different methods can be used to prevent and change cortex-based musings that might activate the amygdala. With preparing, you can adjust your cortex to be less disposed to activate your amygdala. The underlying advance is to see when the cortex is conveying contemplations that might incite tension. Exactly when you become aware of these considerations and their nervousness prompting impacts, you can begin to see them, recognize when they occur, and figure out how to change them.

CHAPTER 5
RECOGNIZING WHERE FEAR AND ANXIETY COMES FROM

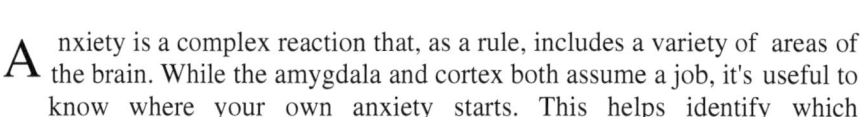

Anxiety is a complex reaction that, as a rule, includes a variety of areas of the brain. While the amygdala and cortex both assume a job, it's useful to know where your own anxiety starts. This helps identify which methodologies will be generally useful in diminishing it. Right now, focus on evaluating whether your anxiety is cortex-based, amygdala-based, or both. You'll also get comfortable with how your own genuine fears and reactions impact you and your life.

Where Does Your Anxiety Begin?

In perspective on earlier parts, you understand that notwithstanding the way that the amygdala is the neurological wellspring of the uneasiness response, making the actual sensations of tension and consistently superseding cortex-based points of view, nervousness doesn't by and large beginning in the amygdala. It can similarly begin in the cortex, with contemplations and mental pictures enacting the amygdala. Assuming you become anxious when you see a growling canine and begin to hyperventilate, that would be amygdala-started uneasiness. Assuming you're pacing fearfully as you imagine a huge call, that would be cortex-started tension. Getting where and how your uneasiness starts will allow you to embrace the best technique to meddle with the procedure.

Remember that when tension beginnings in the amygdala, cortex-based musings, rationale and thinking for instance, don't by and large assist with diminishing nervousness. Amygdala-based anxiety can frequently be recognized by specific attributes; for instance, it appears to originate suddenly, it makes solid physiological reactions, and it appears to be messed up with regards to the circumstance. Right when tension starts in the amygdala, you need to use the language of the amygdala to adjust it. Amygdala-started tension is most enough diminished by the mediations in Chapter 2 of this book, "Accepting Accountability for Your Amygdala-Based Anxiety."

If, of course, you understand that your nervousness began in the cortex, the more

fruitful strategy is to change your appearance to lessen the ensuing amygdala authorization. You'll look into how you can accomplish this in Chapter 3 of the book, "Accepting Accountability for Your Cortex-Based Anxiety." Decreasing the events wherein your cortex causes your amygdala to become started will dispense with your overall tension. The rest of this segment includes relaxed examinations that will help you with surveying and depict your normal tension responses to help you in sorting out where your nervousness starts. You should take note of that these aren't logical assessments; they're basically given to help you with researching your amygdala and cortex-based inclinations.

CORTEX-BASED ANXIETY

We'll start by watching out for uneasiness began by hardware in the cortex. Specific kinds of commencement in the cortex, routinely experienced as contemplations, can in the end make the amygdala authorize the tension response, close by the whole of its disturbing signs. The collections of cortex-based inception are different, yet they all have a comparative expected result: placing you at risk for experiencing tension. The going with assessments will give more information into unquestionably the most essential ways the cortex pathway can begin uneasiness and will help you with recognizing which ones you experience. Ordinarily, people don't give close thought to the specific contemplations occurring in their cortex, so it is fundamental that you become logically cautious and aware of what's happening in your cortex at some irregular moment. By sorting out some way to see different kinds of nervousness inciting cortex works out, you can transform them before they develop into out and out uneasiness. We'll reveal how to do as such in Chapter 3 of the book.

Exercise: Assessing Left Hemisphere–Based Anxiety

As explained in Chapter 3, the left 50% of the half of the globe of the cortex can convey a kind of restless dread that shows up as a tendency to worry about what will happen and check regularly for game plans. With this sort of nervousness, people will overall ruminate or spotlight earnestly on a situation or need to look at a situation over and over.

Read the models underneath and check those that depict you:

- ☐   *I practice potential issue conditions to me, considering various ways things could turn out seriously and how I'll respond.*
- ☐   *I every now and again think about conditions from a prior time and consider*

    ways they might have gone better.
- ☐   *I will more often than not stall out during the time spent considering different ways I could talk with someone about worries or distinctive points.*
- ☐   *Sometimes I can't kill a flood of adverse thinking, and it often keeps me from sleeping.*
- ☐   *I imagine that its calming to contemplate a trouble from different substitute places of view.*
- ☐   *I feel greatly improved when I have a response for a possible trouble, simply in the event that the situation emerges.*
- ☐   *I understand I will more often than not harp on inconveniences, but it's since I'm endeavoring to find explanations for them.*
- ☐   *I experience trouble getting myself to stop considering things that make me anxious.*

If you actually look at a couple of the things above, you may be contributing a ton of energy focusing on upsetting conditions and deriving musings that extend your level of tension. Despite the way that your left hemi-circle may be looking for a reply, a strong focus on potential hardships can start the amygdala. You may be botching various freedoms for uneasiness free minutes by considering issues which may never happen.

The left half of the side of the equator provides us with a part of our by and large mind boggling and significantly made limits, and we individuals couldn't have made the creatively refined world we live in without its commitments. In any case, the pressure and rumination it makes don't offer the response for nervousness. We'll research various ways the left 50% of the mind adds to uneasiness. We'll help you with recognizing unequivocal kinds of perspectives that lead to nervousness, for instance, negativity, stress, obsessions, habitualness, catastrophizing, responsibility, and disgrace, and explain how you can change these idea processes.

The right half of the globe of the cortex grants you to use your imaginative brain to envision events that aren't actually occurring. Imagining disturbing conditions can order the amygdala. The right half of the side of the equator's consideration on nonverbal pieces of human associations, For example, visible presentations, way of talking, or non-verbal correspondence, may take you leap toward decisions about this information. For instance, it's everything except hard to make a super presentation or a sign and expect someone is furious or disillusioned.

Read the assertions under and check any that you experience frequently:

- ☐ *I picture potential issue conditions to me, imagining various ways things could turn out seriously and how others will respond.*
- ☐ *I'm extremely open to the tone of people's voices.*
- ☐ *I can regularly imagine a couple of circumstances that show how a situation could end up being bad for me.*
- ☐ *I will, as a general rule, imagine ways that people will investigate or excuse me.*
- ☐ *I often imagine ways that I might embarrass myself.*
- ☐ *I a portion of the time see pictures of dreadful events happening.*
- ☐ *I rely upon my sense to get what others are feeling and thinking.*
- ☐ *I'm mindful of people's non-verbal correspondence and comprehend circumspect signals.*

If you actually look at a few of the assertions over, your uneasiness may be expanded by a tendency to imagine disturbing circumstances or rely upon normal interpretations of people's appearance that may not be definite. These right-side of the equator based techniques can cause your amygdala to respond like you're in an unsafe situation when no risk exists. An assortment of procedures, including play, exercise, musings, and pictures can be useful for expanding incitation of the left 50% of the cerebrum, delivering good sentiments, and quieting the right half of the hemisphere.

In Chapter 3, we inspected how the translation of events, conditions, and others' responses can provoke tension. Exactly when this occurs, a singular's cortex is making unnecessary nervousness. The tension is being conveyed not by the situation, but by the way where the cortex is translating the situation. To conclude whether your cortex will in general change fair-minded circumstances into wellsprings of uneasiness, read through the summary underneath and check any things that worry you:

- ☐ *I will generally expect the worst.*

☐   *I think I ponder people's comments too literally.*
☐   *I experience trouble enduring the way that I submit mistakes, and I beat myself up   when I do.*
☐   *I regularly don't say 'no' when I ought to, in light of the fact that I'm terrified of baffling people.*
☐   *I will quite often zero in on any blemishes in my appearance.*
☐   *When I experience trouble finding something that I pushed on, I think of it as an analysis.*

Assuming you actually look at a couple of things, consider whether you're contributing a lot of your energy focusing on reflections or activities that keep you trapped in plans that keep up your tension as time goes on and prevent you from getting important time. Over the top considerations can occur without dire practices, but routinely driving forces structure when a singular see that these practices give momentary mitigation from uneasiness. Tragically, notwithstanding the way that the motivations don't help as time goes on, they can be kept up with by the amygdala because of the concise easing from tension that tails them. As such, adjusting to obsessions and motivations commonly requires an approach that destinations the amygdala similarly as the cortex. We'll discuss techniques for overseeing cortex-based obsessions in Chapter 3 and explain show procedures that battle amygdala-filled driving forces in Chapter 8.

Since you've recognized cortex-based purposes behind your tension, we'll help you with assessing your tendency toward amygdala-started uneasiness. As an update, at whatever point you feel tension or dread, the amygdala is incorporated. Regardless, the going with assessments will help you with zeroing in on encounters where your uneasiness response started in the amygdala. At the point when you know the early phase, you can pick advances toward that will best control your nervousness. Assuming the hardware in the actual amygdala is what begun your uneasiness, methods that emphasis on the cortex will be useless.

To choose Assuming the amygdala or the cortex began a specific tension response, you need to think about what was happening before you began to experience nervousness. Assuming you were focusing on explicit musings, that recommends that your tension began in the cortex. If, once more, you feel that a specific article, region, or situation immediately evoked a nervousness response, the amygdala will undoubtedly be the start stage.

Exercise: Assessing Your Experience of Unexplained Anxiety

At the moment that your uneasiness has all the earmarks of being unexplained or begins out of nowhere and you can't find any legitimate avocation for it, your amygdala is

probably the explanation. You may truly say, "I essentially have no idea why I have this impression; it doesn't check out," since none of your contemplations or current experiences legitimize the inclination. As we've seen, the amygdala habitually responds without your having any conscious thoughtfulness regarding what's happening, and the responses it makes are consistently astounding.

Read the going with declarations, which reflect unexplained tension, and check any that worry you:

- ☐ *Sometimes my heart pounds for reasons unknown.*
- ☐ *When I visit others, I as frequently as conceivable need to get back, in spite of the way that things are going fine.*
- ☐ *I routinely don't feel accountable for my passionate reactions.*
- ☐ *I can't explain why I react the way where I do by and large.*
- ☐ *I have sudden floods of uneasiness that seem to seem unexpectedly.*
- ☐ *I essentially don't feel extraordinary taking off to explicit spots; in any case, I don't have a valid justification for feeling that way.*
- ☐ *I regularly feel panicky with no notice.*
- ☐ *I can't perceive the triggers of my anxiety.*

As we've noted, you probably won't move toward the amygdala's recollections. As needs be, the point at which your amygdala reacts you may not get what it's reacting to or why. The elevating news is, regardless, when you're not sure why your amygdala is responding, you can investigate a wide combination of systems to assist with calming your amygdala and redo it.

Exercise: Assessing Your Experience of Rapid Physiological Responding

At the moment that the amygdala is the wellspring of your uneasiness, you will undoubtedly have unmistakable physiological changes as one of the important signs of your nervousness. Before you have the chance to think or even totally process the situation, you might experience a beating heart, sweating, and a dry mouth. Since the amygdala is unequivocally wired to animate the thoughtful sensory system, start muscles, and release adrenaline into the circulatory framework, having physiological appearances as the essential sign of uneasiness is a good pointer that you're overseeing amygdala-based anxiety.

Read the going with articulations, which reflect speedy physiological reaction, and check any that worry you:

- ☐   *I observe that my heart is dashing regardless, when there's no undeniable explanation.*
- ☐   *I can go from feeling calm to being in an all out alarm shockingly fast.*
- ☐   *I suddenly can't get my breathing mind-set to feel right.*
- ☐   *Sometimes I feel insecure or similarly as I nod off, and these feelings arise rapidly.*
- ☐   *My stomach falters and I feel nauseous immediately.*
- ☐   *I become aware of my heart since I have torment or inconvenience in my chest.*
- ☐   *I start sweating without laboring.*
- ☐   *I do not know what comes over me. I essentially start shuddering all of a sudden.*

If you checked countless these assertions, which reflect strong and quick physiological responding, your tension might start in reactivity of the amygdala. Exactly when you experience such responses, you might acknowledge that a genuine danger is accessible. Regardless, your amygdala could be reacting to a trigger that is certainly not a careful pointer of hazard, so recall that an opinion of risk doesn't actually show the proximity of a risk. You can use these physiological responses as a sign that you ought to use the frameworks proposed Chapter 2 of this book.

Exercise: Assessing Your Experience of Unplanned Aggressive Feelings or Behavior

A tendency toward aggression relies upon the battle part of the battle, flight, or freeze response. However a couple of individuals need to pull out and avoid conflicts or compromising conditions, others will overall have forceful responses. Unexpectedly feeling compromised can make them leaned to shock and erupting at others. This strong response, which has its fundamental establishments in the cautious thought of the amygdala, is especially normal for people with post-horrendous pressure disorder.

Read the going with articulations, which reflect spontaneous forceful opinions or lead, and check any that worry you:

- ☐   *I burst out of nowhere in explicit circumstances.*
- ☐   *I regularly need to design something physical for express my disappointment.*
- ☐   *I strike out and later comprehend that my response was unnecessarily solid.*
- ☐   *I snap at others with little notice.*

- ☐ *I feel that I'm good for hurting someone when I'm under pressure.*
- ☐ *I would rather not erupt at people, yet I can't resist.*
- ☐ *Family people and associates know to be cautious around me.*
- ☐ *When I've been vexed, I've broken or thrown objects.*

If you checked a couple of these assertions, which give signs of restless enmity, your amygdala's attempts to sanction a forceful response, but you can apply control by the manner in which you direct your direct. Customary actual exercise can assist with really taking a look at this kind of responding and taking an energetic walk around get away from a compromising situation can assist with satisfying the drive to make prompt move.

Exercise: Assessing Your Experience of Inability to Think Clearly

At the moment that you get yourself fretful just as inadequate to focus or facilitate the point of convergence of your thought, this is a strong marker of amygdala-based tension. Exactly when the amygdala steps in, it assumes control over the attentional control of the cortex and accepts accountability. Exactly when you experience this amygdala-based control of your psyche, you'll feel unsuitable to control your considerations. Remember, according to a formative perspective the amygdala's ability to clutch control when it perceives danger assisted our eliminated antecedents with persevering. Thusly, the amygdala has held this breaking point. Regardless, it's both annoying and disillusioning to unexpectedly lose the ability to pick what to focus on or consider.

Read the going with explanations, which reflect a failure to think obviously, and check any that worry you:

- ☐ *When I'm feeling under tension, my brain goes clear and I can't think.*
- ☐ *I understand that when I'm fretful, I can't focus on what I have to do.*
- ☐ *When I get restless, I can't concentrate well overall.*
- ☐ *When I'm being shouted at, I can't imagine a reaction.*
- ☐ *When I feel panicky, it's difficult for me to focus on what I need to do.*
- ☐ *Even when I endeavor to calm down, it's hard for me to occupy myself from how my body is feeling.*
- ☐ *When I'm scared, on occasion I draw a flat out clear with regards to what I should do straightaway.*

If you checked a couple of these assertions, you may as frequently end up in conditions where you have a feebleness to think. The associations from the amygdala to the cortex can affect how thought is composed, and evidence suggests that people who experience raised degrees of uneasiness regularly have additional weak relationship from the cortex to the amygdala (Kim et al. 2011). Cortex-based methodology for adjusting to tension are routinely not significant when the amygdala is activated. A piece of the strategies discussed later, for instance, full breathing or loosening up, will be valuable regardless, when your perspectives are limited by institution of the amygdala.

Printed in Great Britain
by Amazon